Dr. Francesco Contarin

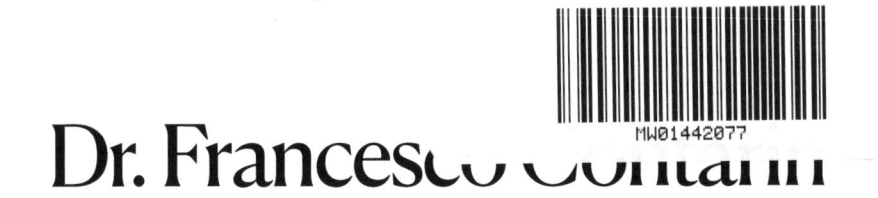

Embarazada después de los 35'

© Dr. Francesco Contarin

Francesco Contarin
301 Altara Ave. Coral Gables, Fl. 33146 USA
www.contarin.net

ISBN: 9798378183531

Créditos: Algunas imágenes de esta obra son propiedad de sus respectivos autores. Tomadas de freepik.com y de unsplash.com

gps

booksurge.

PostScript Error

date	2023/03/25
time	07:34:38
printer	CAE36320-10
Error identification	ioerror
Offending Command	--image--
Operand Stack	Top -dict-
Execution Stack	Top { _Filte Top-1 -file- Top-2 { --dis Top-3 -- @ab Top-4 { --clea --exch
Dictionary Stack	Top -dict- Top-1 -dict- Top-2 -dict- Top-3 -dict- Top-4 //userc

Stray Tarot
How to Survive as a Tarot Reader

Pitisci

Stray Tarot – How to Survive aa a Tarot Reader   Copyright © 2018 by Vincent Pitisci

All rights reserved. No part of this book may be reproduced in any form, except brief excerpts for purpose of review without written permission from the author.

CreateSpace Independent Publishing Platform

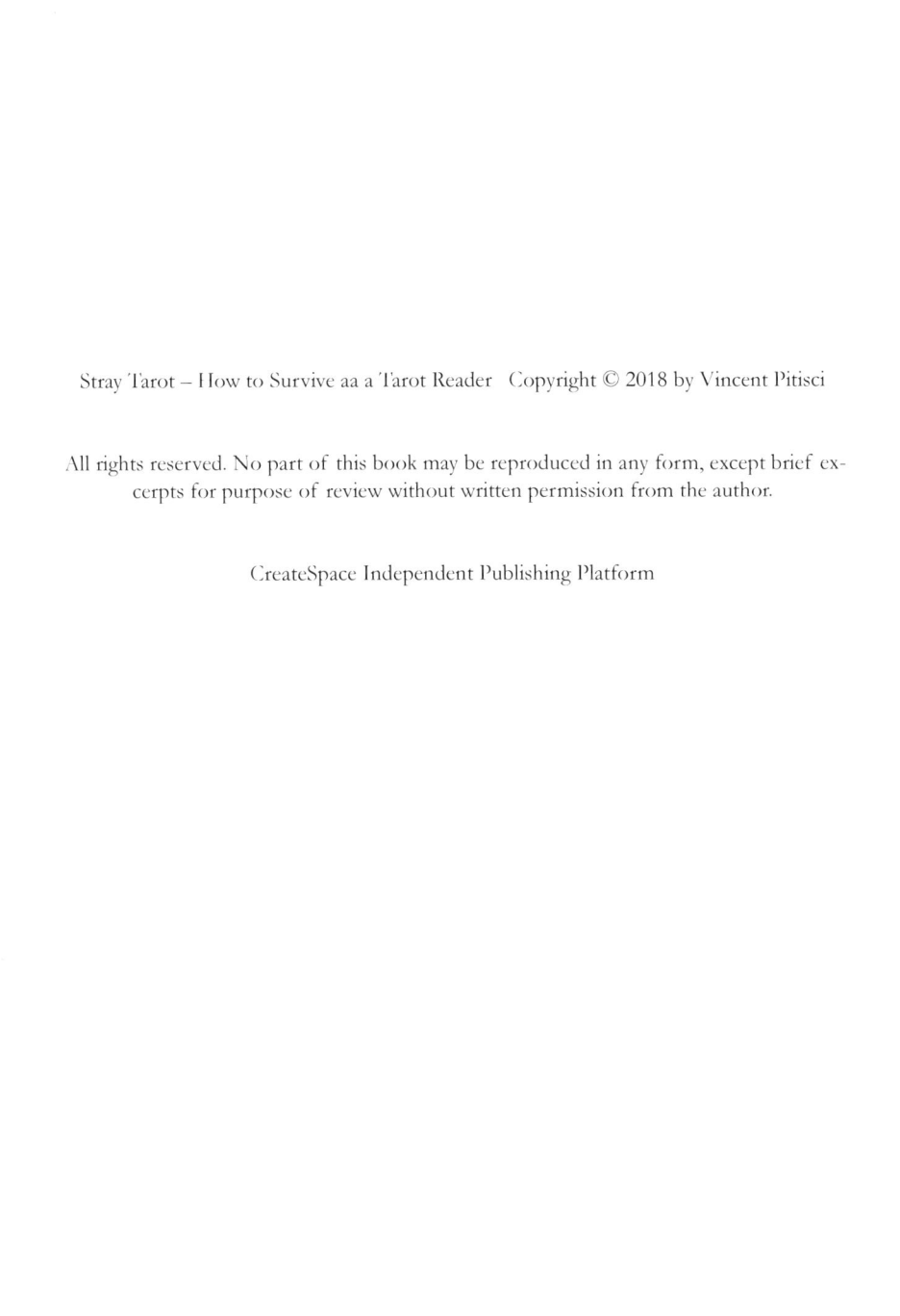

Dedication

To the ghost of Tom Joad

Contents

Acknowledgments

Preface – 200 miles north

Introduction 13

Chapter 1. Laying the groundwork................................19

Chapter 2. Being a House Reader..................................25

Chapter 3. Fairs/Festivals and other big events.............29

Chapter 4. Phone Readings – A Key Asset...................41

Chapter 5. About Reading Paying Clients....................47

Chapter 6. Little Bits of Insight....................................53

Chapter 7. Who am I?...61

Chapter 8. Some Tarot Reading Stories........................67

Chapter 9. Other Professional Thoughts.......................79

Chapter 10. How to Approach Professional Readings............87

Chapter 11. Reading the Tarot Fluently........................93

Chapter 12. Why the Tarot Works................................99

ACKNOWLEDGMENTS

Lawrence Howard Clairvoyant/Astral Traveler who I first met in 1956
Frank Shoeman Clairvoyant/Occultist who I first met around 1957
Lillian Hunter Clairvoyant/Psychic who I first met around 1958
The Theosophical Society in Wheaton,IL since 1956
The Rosicrucian Order Nefertiti Lodge Chicago since 1956

Betty Livingston professional Palmist who I first met around 1993
The Amazing Leonard Psychic/Tarot reader who I first met around 1993
To Monica.....the good witch I've known since 1993
Professor Drew who I first met in 1993

Mort Shanker Psychic Fairs – first read professionally in 1993
Angels Forever Bookstore – first read professionally in 1994
Carol's Crystal Castle – first read professionally in 1996
The Inner Eye Bookstore – first read professionally in 1996
Unseen Insights – first read professionally in 1997
Sanctuary Crystals – first read professionally in 2001
The Quest Bookstore – first read professionally in 2010

and to all the other people and places I just can't recall.

Thanks!

Preface

200 miles north

We have a few friends up in Green Bay, WI, who we have read for in their New Age book store from time to time. Over the years we have always remained friends.

Now that Lynda and I are back living in Chicago, IL, it has been awhile since we have gotten together with our friends up north.

We decided to have me come up for a day and read at their store as a guest reader. The day was set for a Saturday from 10am till 5pm.
I got up that morning at 4am and got on the road by 5:30am with all of my things needed for the day. I got there at 9:50am and my first reading walked in the door right at 10am. The appointments were all made in advance and I was booked solid for the day, 12 half-hour readings with an hour break from 1pm till 2pm.

All went well and the readings were kept right on time.
The owners made their end look easy and handled everything just like the pros they are.

I handled my end making it look easy as well, and all the readings were good and right on time with no setbacks. Smooth as silk.

Afterwards we closed shop and stopped off for a few drinks and talked old times.

Lynda and I have many memories long past with them and a lot of the conversation was about how it was too bad Lynda had another commitiment in Chicago and couldn't make the trip with me.

They took me for a prime rib dinner at a nice place and then we went out for more entertainment. The drinks kept coming and my wallet was not allowed to come out of my pocket.

At 10pm we decided to go home. I was to spend the night at their place and the room was set. We sat in their kitchen still talking old times the four of us had as we were having a nightcap.

Then the phone rang and it was a friend of theirs telling them to meet up at another pub. So we got in their car and went out again for more punishment till 1am.

We went back to their place and had a nightcap again at their kitchen table.

As the picture shows, the cat liked me by then, making himself right at home on my shoulders.

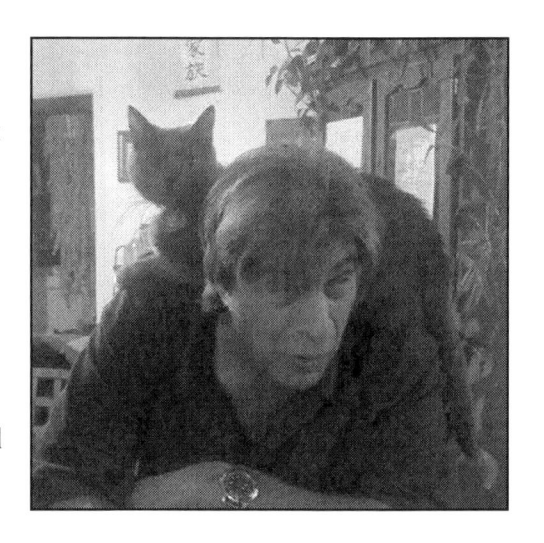

Went to bed around 3am (don't know if the cat came with me or not) and got up at 7am. They made me breakfast and the morning was nice. Good friends.

I said good-bye at 9:30 and hit the highway back to Chicago.
Four hours on a peaceful Sunday morning. Traffic is light at that time of day.

Walked in the door at 1:30 or so and Lynda was there to ask how it all went.

I pulled out a pocket full of twenties and said it went real good.

Life is great!

Introduction

Over the past 25 years I have taught many students how to read the Tarot. After they have learned the cards they always have the same question.

"How do I get started as a reader?"

Many books are written on how to use the Tarot cards. But I haven't come across anything written on what to do after you learn the cards. You wanna read professionally? How do you get started? There is no manual out there telling you how to be a pro reader. Not that I'm aware of anyway. I am closer to the end of this wonderful journey than I am to the beginning of it, so I felt it was time to share with you how I did it.

I don't feel there is any reason to hide anything about it. I made a living as a card reader and I loved every minute of it. In these pages you will hear how I did it. You will also see that you can do it as well.

Is it really possible to earn a living as a card reader? Yes it is. I know because I already did it. I was never late with the rent and I live happily. The best way to go about this is buffet style, not one main course, In other words a little of this and a little of that.

I've done house parties, festivals, read out of many New Age book stores, coffee houses, psychic hot lines, and boutiques just to name a few ideas for you. I do phone readings as well. One avenue will help the other. They all start to get intertwined after time.

As you move on in your quest you will meet others on this path as well. And exchanging ideas with each other is another part of this wonderful experience.

What will you need?
A willingness to take a risk, no fear of failure, and owning up to it when it happens. A sincere feeling of wanting to help guide others in their quests through life. And staying honest and above board if you are in it for the long haul.

There is one other thing. A passion to be a reader. Oh, and yes, a deck of 78 cards known as the Tarot. The rest is all down hill......Well sorta.

There is a difference between art and work. If you make a living as a Tarot reader you are an artist. Your palette is 78 cards and your canvas is any table you place those mysterious cards on.

Your talent is your confidence with a deck of Tarot cards. Also having a passion for the unknown and what's possible.

This book is not written because I'm trying to achieve something more. I already did it. I just wanted to share with you how I did it. How I got through it. Do I have any regrets? No. I feel wonderful about my accomplishments in the craft. I've come to know many other readers over the years as well. Some were full time readers, some were part time readers but it has always been fun to be part of that whole thing and I hope that I helped make it fun for them as well.

I would say half the readers I started with 25 years ago are no longer with us, but their spirits will be with me as long as I'm around. The other half are still going strong as readers. Once you start, you won't be able to give it up. The experience is just too good to leave behind.

Another asset for me as a reader was my life partner. Her name is Lynda. She is just plain psychic and didn't need cards although she would lay them out if you liked. That was 1993.

We met at one of my classes I was holding at a New Age bookstore. The owner invited her to attend. Lynda was this tall beautiful psychic with wild *Stevie Nicks* type blond hair. So I asked her if I could give her a call after the class. She said yes. I called her that night and saw her every night after that. We were hitting it off. A few weeks later I took her to a Chinese restaurant (women like Chinese food) and I asked her if she would like to become partners as professional psychics. She said yes again. Two yeses in a row! She knew a lot more of the pro readers at that time than I did and they all wanted her to read with them.

I remember Marlena, who held some big psychic fairs in the area, really wanted Lynda on her crew. But Marlena wasn't interested in me at all. Lynda wouldn't do it unless it was both of us. We were partners. So we never read for Marlena's fairs. But we sure read everywhere else, all over Chicago.

Lynda had the contacts and I hung on to her coat tail for the ride. We were a team. The best team in Chicago.

I asked her to marry me three years later on the karaoke at my company Xmas party at the printing company I worked at. She accepted!

That was 1996. I left the printing industry for good in 2005 and I've just read cards since then. The marriage wasn't going well so in 2007 we divorced but we still remained loving partners and we still saw each other every day.

We were divorced for 10 years but the divorce wasn't working out too well either. It takes work to maintain a good divorce. Today we discuss ending the divorce now and then although we have worked on it so hard. We might just get remarried and forget the whole thing ever happened. If I consult the cards on it they seem to say *"Don't put me in the middle of this!"*

I know she still cares for me. (How could you not!) I feel that I am in Lynda's top ten as far as past boyfriends go. Probably somewhere around number 7 or 8, but the top ten for sure.

So I can say that my whole professional career as a reader was with my life partner Lynda. This made it easier to do. Actually I don't think I could have done it without her by my side. But we do know a lot of psychics that did it alone. Either way, I know you can do it too.

As with any career there is a period of time needed to learn the trade. There is no diploma or degree for intuitive thinking.
Your college is the world itself, and how you interact with it as you follow your passion.

So whether you read part time, full time, with a partner or without one, this book will show you how.

What is Prediction?

Any time we have a question concerning something we are attempting to accomplish, we look for an answer in the future. Something that needs to still be done. That means a future action. That is a prediction. A prediction is a statement concerning what is to come. Many predictions require action to take place. If we do this action – this result will happen. Prediction.

Society relies on many predictions. Stock market and weather reports are two common ones. Marketing strategies are another. The FBI might make a prediction based on criminal behavior when seeking a Most Wanted suspect. Point spreads on the weekly football games are predictions. We call the seer an odds maker but they are predicting an answer just the same.

Jimmy the Greek was probably the most widely known, televised odds maker in the game of football. My guess is he was only about 65% correct on his predictions. He was famous for being one of the best. Today Nostradamus is still considered a renowned mystic for his ability to predict the future. We still follow his quatrains. Many of his predictions never came to pass. He's probably around 65% accurate as well.

The Tarot card reader also predicts the future. The more accurate your predictions are, the more business you will have. Any reader who says they are 100% accurate probably needs to have their doctor adjust their medication.

Some clients will stay with you as their reader until you are wrong one time. Then they seek another reader to take your place. How long you keep them as a client will depend on your consistency of accuracy. Other clients will stay with you no matter how many times you're incorrect. They just like you as their reader. The rest are in between the two.

A Tarot card reading is all about finding new ideas, seeing things that weren't seen before you and your client sat down with the cards. Then, if those new ideas work sometime down the road – in the future – you have done a successful reading.

Life is full of challenges. If you can steer a client in a positive direction that they didn't see before and that new direction pans out well as a solution, you have accomplished a successful reading. You will have also gained a steady client for future readings. You will have earned their trust.

As a professional, you will want to gain a client's trust and have them believe you might be able to see a different angle to their present challenge, something they didn't see by themselves. But together, you and her were able to see new light on a question asked. An answer. A solution.

You become the answer man. And if your answers work, you will have them come back for other answers in the future, when they need them.

You will keep them as a client as long as your batting average is higher than most other input and advice they get.

A reader is a like a lighthouse and the client is like a ship at sea. You guide them into a safe and secure harbor. And when they feel a need for direction again, they will be searching for your guiding light in this wonderful and amazing sea of life.

As a reader, you not only experience life. You witness it in others exciting journey through it. Some are wonderful. Some are desperate. Some are sad. Some are happy. But all are magnificent.

1. Laying the groundwork

Having things in order before you take this plunge will be to your advantage. Make this move when finances are in good order. Not being in any serious debt will be good for you as well. Whenever you start a new type of business you will be vulnerable at first. So being in a good financial position is best. What this really means is not being in debt, and hopefully having a few dollars stored away to fall back on to begin with. A few months rent in the bank can really be helpful too.

HEALTHCARE BENEFITS:
Many people have said they would like to start working for themselves but can't because they would lose their healthcare benefits. Now that has finally changed. You can get healthcare insurance based on your income through the Affordable Care Act. Go to HEALTHCARE.GOV and you will see your options available to you.

Yes we have finally evolved to the point where you have the right to health care without working for a big company! Just like the rest of the world! This is great news!

Go to HEALTHCARE.GOV
It is your right.

Some advantages to being a professional Tarot reader are there is no overhead. No cost. No store front to rent out. The only thing needed is a deck of Tarot cards and a place to read them. No set up time at fairs, events and festivals either. So you can travel light with no need to order or carry around any cumbersome merchandise.

Stuff on your Things to Do list:
Have something to hand out to people you meet. Business cards are great but anything with your name and phone number on it will work. Some readers will have book marks printed with their contact information on them.

As long as you have something to hand to people you meet up with. For me, a simple business card with your name, cell phone number, email and your website if you have one is all you need.

I use VISTAPRINT.COM for all of my printed material.
They are easy to use and will help you if you have any questions about what you want printed.

Finding places to work out of:
The best way to start out is working at a New Age type bookstore. Have the bookstore schedule you to be there one or two days every week. If clients know you are there every Wednesday and Friday, for example, it helps them to set up another reading with you at that store.

Being at a certain coffee house once a week is good as well to get your name out there. Many coffee houses would be happy to have you there. Talk to the owner and set up a day during the week that you would be there. Go there on your scheduled day every week. Sit there with a cup of coffee and read a book with a modest table tent type sign that says

PSYCHIC READINGS   or   TAROT READINGS
$20 – 15 MINUTES $20 – 15 MINUTES

Whatever is your personal preference.
If people know you are there, let's say, every Wednesday from 6 till 9pm the word will get out. It will probably take some time before people realize you are there every week, but after awhile you will start to get people coming up to your table and asking about a reading with you.

Maybe the coffee house will put something in the window advertising you as well. Another helpful thing is if you can supply some printed material about you that the owner can keep on the counter as hand-outs.

Annual fairs and festivals are a great place for the card reader. They are also times of the year you can count on to bring in business. OctoberFest, and The Fourth of July are two good examples. If you see an event for OctoberFest and there is a Ferris wheel and carnival, it is a good bet for you.

Carnivals are usually there three or four days, which means the festival will be there the same amount of time. A three or four day fair will cost you a vendor's fee but it should still be worth the effort. If you do an annual festival like this and you like it, make sure you keep the contact information so you can reschedule again for next year.

Events you do annually allow you to anticipate business coming ahead. Having a few of these events scheduled during the year should work well for you. It's money you can count on to come during the year.

Another good source to network business is lounges. Many lounges have what's called Ladies Night. This might be a monthly event or maybe semi-annual depending on the owner. Here they will have a few vendors set up selling their wares - purses, jewelry, and things like that. You can be one of the vendors, doing Tarot readings.

Around the holiday season you can go to businesses who might have Xmas or New Years Eve parties. Believe it or not, you can find a company party that is interested in having you there. If it works out, remember to get someone's contact info and try to schedule again for the following year as well.

Company picnics in the summer can also bring you work. If you find any out there, see what they think about having you as a reader.

Valentines Day at big name clothes stores like Macy's can be something to look into as well. They will set you up like a "see Santa" thing as the "Love Psychic". This type of thing is best for the women readers.

Make sure people know you do house parties and coporate events. Some can turn into business that becomes steady, annual events you can count on every year.

Some local pubs love having a Psychic Night and you can become a regular there as well.

Most flea markets don't allow psychic readers to set up shop in my area but if you can get into one, do it. Doing 10 minutes for $20 works well for that type of setting. The readings are light and breezy and can attract people to seek you out for a more serious reading later on. Again make sure that whoever you read gets your contact information.

So there are many places that could be interested in having you as a Tarot reader. These are just some of the ones I've used successfully. It really just comes down to you taking the initiative and asking.

Remember that it's a matter of getting your name out there. That means having people talk with you. This is why I feel it's important to have a bright image of who you are.

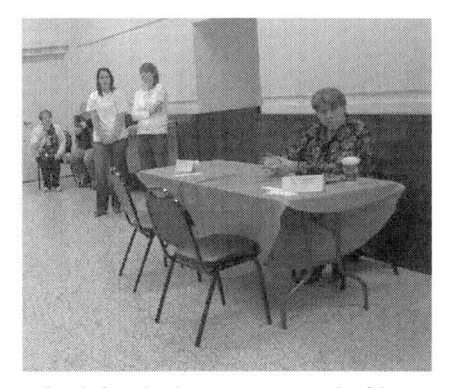

Just before the doors open at a vendor fair.

A dark looking person can make people shy away from them in many of these settings, especially as a card reader. That craft has a reputation of being shady.

Present yourself as someone who is optimistic and has nothing to hide. A white witch look will get you more business than a black witch look. And that goes for your little dog, too!

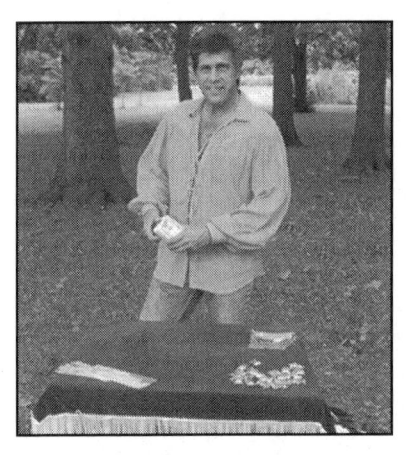

An outside event in 2005

A Tarot reader holding a class at a coffee house.

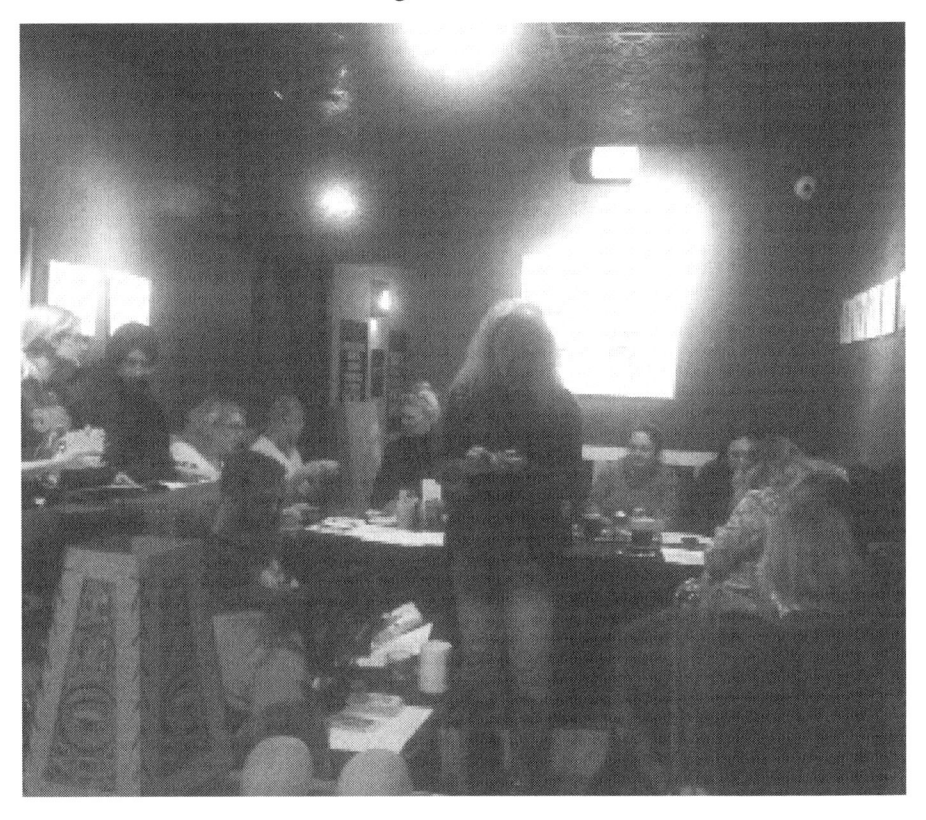

2. Being a House Reader

Many places will have what's called a House Reader. This is a person who does readings on scheduled days during the week at the store. These will mostly be what I call New Age bookstores. New Age bookstores usually sell candles, incense, books on astrology, tarot cards, the paranormal, and other spiritual items. They might offer classes on these types of subjects as well.

Most stores like this will also have readings available to the public given by house readers. These are readers the store sponsors and advertises. If you are a house reader at one of these places you would be assigned specific days that you read on, let's say Wednesday and Saturday.

You would be at the store, ready to read anyone the store has scheduled that day for a reading. The store makes all the appointments and collects all the money. At the end of the day you would be paid a percentage of that day's purse. The store takes a percentage of the money from those readings, usually 25% to 50% percent, depending on the store.

Stores will compete for good readers by keeping their percentage of the purse lower than their competition, hoping to attract the best readers. Stores hope that you will bring in a following and drum up more business for the store. You hope to increase your customer base by meeting new clients that visit that store.

Working at a New Age type store will probably require you to do an interview reading with the owner to make sure that they like the way you read. If they ask you for an interview-type reading, they like you already. You'll do fine.

After you are there awhile you will start to get regulars that come to see you. You will start to acquire a following. Make sure you give everyone you read at the store your business card and tell them they can always see you there at the store but they can also call you directly anytime for a phone reading. The money from phone readings is all yours; the store does not get anything for that.

The store only gets money for the readings done at the store. This is important to remember. Once people have had a few face-to-face readings with you they feel more comfortable getting phone readings with you. Phone readings are very convenient for both you and the client. The chapter on phone readings will go into this more.

If you do work a store like this you might be asked to do a simple or basic one-day class on your craft. This would be set up and scheduled and advertised by the store. So if you become a house reader plan on opportunities to also do some classes.

Classes can be fun and they bring in extra money as well. If 6 people sign up for a one-day, three-hour class on Tarot cards and the class costs $50, that would be $300. The percentage sould be the same as you get for reading there. Let's say the store takes 25%. That would be $225 for you and $75 for the store. Not bad for just talking about Tarot cards while sitting there sipping on a Starbucks coffee.

This is a good place to practice doing classes on the Tarot. Once you get good at it you could do classes at other places like public libraries, or special interest night classes at schools or anywhere that might be interested. I enjoy the classroom setting and look forward to classes when I have them. You learn a lot by teaching as well.

Teaching the Tarot can actually make you a better reader, so think about trying to do a class at a New Age bookstore some day.
Class sizes will vary from one scheduled class to another. I've had as many as 30 people sign up for one of my classes. I've had a little as one person sign up, too. So you never know.

If only one or two people sign up for your class and the class is advertised as a 3 hour class you can cut the class short. You can say that seeing the class is so small everything can be covered a lot quicker on a more one-on-one basis. Therefore the class is only an hour-and-a-half, not three hours long.

New Age bookstores are still one of my favorite places to work. The clients that visit the store will probably be people who have had readings with the other house readers at that store as well.

You will be compared to the other readers and feedback will be given to the owner. Everyone reads differently, so some clients will love the way you read and some might like the way another reader at that store reads better than your reading. Don't take it personally.

New Age bookstores are starting to fade away to some degree. In the 1970's thru the 90's they were big. They were the only place you could get books on those mysterious subjects. But today all bookstores have material available on astrology, tarot cards, spirits guides, and anything else dealing with metaphysics.

Today we have the internet and Amazon. The only thing the New Age bookstore still has that has not been followed by big chain stores is semi precious stones, and house readers. So when people want to get out and visit the store, buy a few special stones, maybe some incense, a book or two, and get a reading, they come to that special New Age bookstore.

3. Festivals, Fairs and other big events

Festivals and fairs will cost you a vendor's fee. Prices will vary but it should be about $50 to $100 per day depending on the size of the festival. A festival I'm currently doing now is Friday through Sunday, noon till midnight all three days. The cost to be a vendor at this event is $450 - a little high priced but we still do it and it works well for us. Electric hook-ups are included. I have done this event for about 12 years now and it's a good fair for me. Splitting the cost with another reader works good here.

I feel the best way to look into investing in being a vendor at a particular annual event is to go there; see the sights first and plan for the following year. If the event is from a Friday to a Sunday, the busiest time will be Saturday evening. The slowest time will be Friday during the day as many people are still at work. So walk through the place and feel it out. Ask a few of the vendors how things are going. They will usually be more than happy to tell you how business is doing.

Watch to see if people are buying things at the booths there. How busy is the midway? By 7 or 8 o'clock it should be very crowded and difficult to walk through. That's a good sign.

Some events will have a parade go though the fair grounds. This would usually take place on a Sunday during the day and might last for a few hours. Parades are bad for business as no one is buying anything at that time. Everyone is just watching the parade going by. So parades are bad for vendors but fun to watch.

If you do decide to be a vendor, ask not to be assigned a spot too close to the sound stage. It would be hard to read over the loud music. If another vendor is selling jewelry, pendants, and things compatible to your services it would be a perfect place for you to be placed next to. The people running the fair will usually be helpful trying to fit you in somewhere that will work well for you.

It's not uncommon for psychic readers to be a vendor. If you see a psychic booth there already, watch them to see how they're doing. If they are slow, look at the booth and see what you would do differently. Many psychic reading booths are bare of scenery. Just a table, two chairs and the reader sitting there with a deck of cards. That doesn't work well.

Most events will not allow two vendors selling the same thing. So if the place already has a psychic vendor booth they probably will not want another one there and they will tell you that. Most places will also honor steady vendors that have been there for a few years. So if the psychic vendor has been there for three or four years they have the place locked in. But if the psychic vendor is there for the first time they might not be interested in coming back next year, especially if they aren't doings things well. That means you can get in there next year and become the psychic vendor booth for that event. Then you are the one locked in for the following years!

If you do an event and you like it, make sure you call the place afterwards and tell them you want to be there next year and ask when you can buy your space. The sooner you buy it, the more secure you become as the one who will be there next year. So lock it in early. After a few years they know you by name and if someone calls to be a psychic vendor they tell them they already have one....You!

Many psychic booths have the readers far in the back of the tent in a dark area. Mysterious kinda atmosphere. To me this is a mistake and people will be curious but afraid to go in there. And that means no business for you. I feel having the readers set up right in front in full view works best. It also creates curiosity as people walk by seeing others getting a reading. They will stop and watch, creating a crowd of people around your booth. That's good for business.

Keep the tent bright and have a nice banner in front so people know right away what you do. Our banner just says "PSYCHIC READINGS" and spans the whole front of the tent. We had the banner made through VISTAPRINT.COM. We also have a sign in front showing the price and amount of time the reading will be. Our signs say
"PSYCHIC READINGS $20 – 10 MINUTES"

We used to do $20 for 15 minutes but as time went on prices went up. Then the going rate went to $25 for 15 minutes. Making change was a real pain. So we went back to $20 and just reduced the time to 10 minutes instead of 15 minutes.

What type of tent:
You will want to purchase what's called a canopy tent. They are also known as gazebo tents. These types of tents have no walls, only a roof. They can be purchased from most department stores like Walmart, Target, Sears and places like that. They will run you around $100 and are easy to set up and take down. They come in 12 ft, 10 ft and 8 ft.

Most events you will see have spaces offered of 10 ft so don't get a 12 ft tent. Get either a 10 ft or an 8 ft. Either will work fine for two readers. If you have three readers or more you will want to get the 10 ft size. In many cases your neighbors will be positioned right next to you, to the foot.

Take the time to know the tent so you can put it up and take it down easily. Taking one down can have different buttons then putting it up so learn both before you go. You don't want to be trying to figure out how to take down your tent at midnight, in the dark on a Sunday night. The makers of these tents have different ways they work. But they are simple to use once you know them.

At night I lower the tent all the way down. It will usually go down to about 4 ft high. This helps keep your tent safe during a bad storm. High winds can bend the frame. If a bad storm comes while you are there and high winds are prevalent, you might want to close shop and lower your tent down a little until things settle down. Just sit tight under your tent and wait it out.

Reading cards on windy days:
If you do any type of event outside you have to fight with the wind.
You lay out your cards and a gust of wind blows your cards off your table. One way around that is to go to the hardware store and buy about a dozen good sized washers. Lay a washer on each card in the spread to keep them on the table. One caution – washers will scratch your cards but it's just part of the wear and tear your deck will go through.

Tables and chairs:

For two readers it's easy enough. Two card tables work fine. But if you have three readers all sitting in a row up front in a 10ft tent you need a different set up. We use two identical folding tables. Two folding tables 4.5ft to 5ft long side by side will allow three readers to sit side by side right in the front of the tent. Put a table cloth over the two tables so that the center reader does not have to deal with the crack between the two tables.

I use folding chairs for the potential clients to sit on. They are only sitting for ten minutes. For the readers I use a more comfortable lawn chair. I have a set of four matching lawn chairs. This type of chair is light weight and as a set, they stack into each other, saving space while packing them into your vehicle.

The Midway is the term used to describe the main walkway of the traffic at the festival.

The Midway

Two Reader set-up

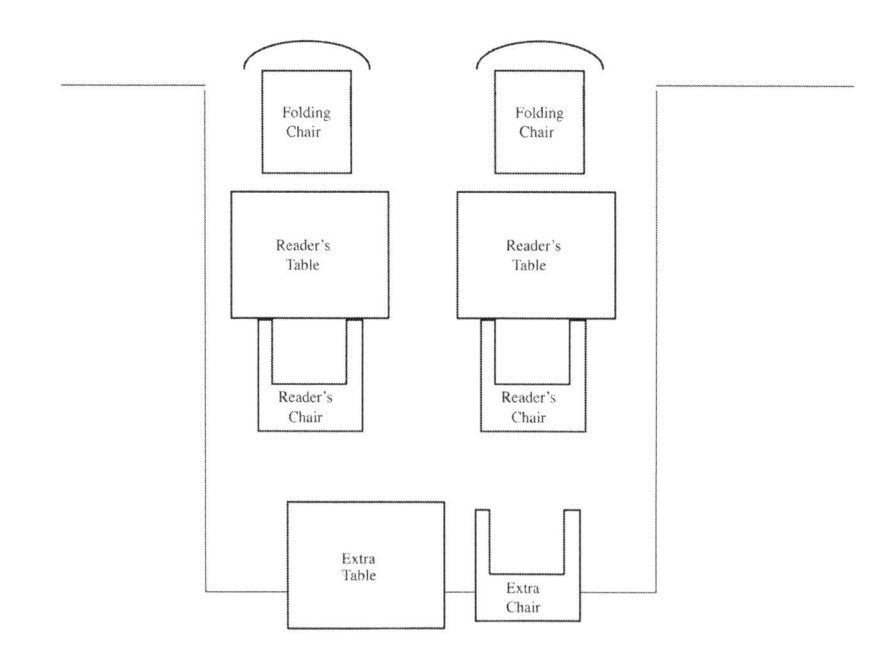

The Midway

Three Reader set-up

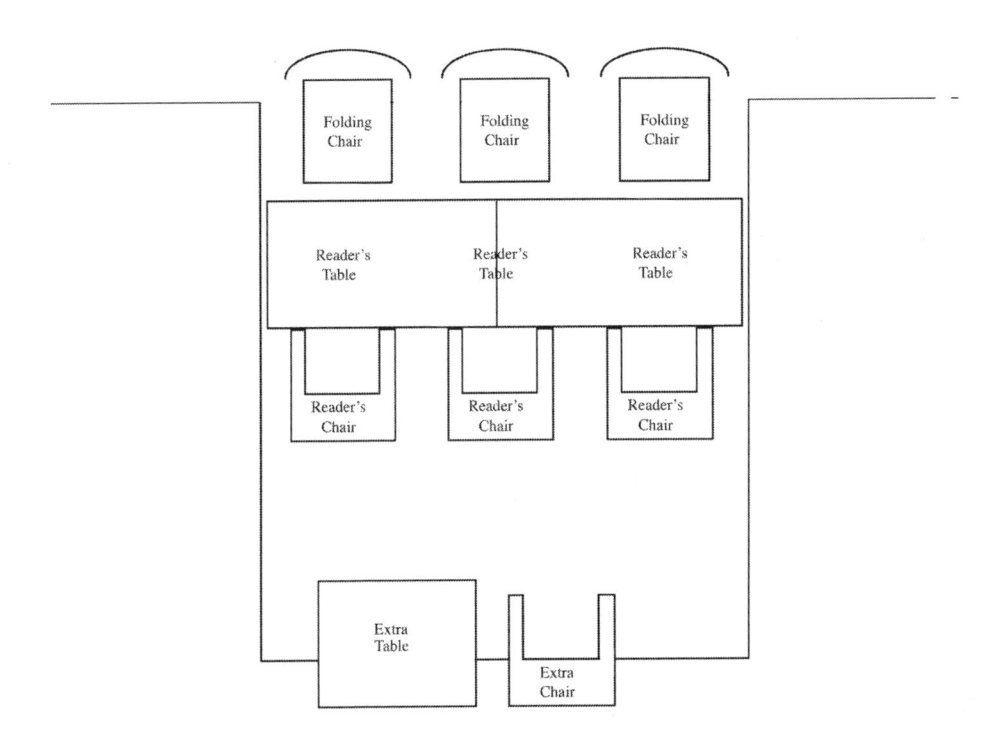

```
       ┌──────┐  ┌──────┐  ┌──────┐
       │Folding│  │Folding│  │Folding│
       │ Chair │  │ Chair │  │ Chair │
       └──────┘  └──────┘  └──────┘
     ┌─────────────────────────────────┐
     │ Reader's    Reader's   Reader's │
     │  Table       Table      Table   │
     └───┬────────────┬───────────┬────┘
         │            │           │
       ┌─┴──┐      ┌──┴─┐      ┌──┴─┐
       │Reader's│  │Reader's│  │Reader's│
       │ Chair │   │ Chair │   │ Chair │
       └──────┘    └──────┘    └──────┘



         ┌──────────────┐
         │              │  ┌────┐
         │    Extra     │  │    │
         │    Table     │  │Extra│
         │              │  │Chair│
         └──────────────┘  └────┘
```

Other extras:
Lights to hang on your tent at night, extension cord to reach the power generator. Power strip to plug lights into. Maybe a fan for hot days. You want to keep in mind that you will have to pack all of your things into one vehicle when you leave Sunday night. When you have a hundred vendors all driving to their booth at the same time you will not be able to get more than one vehicle to your area to pack up. That means the tent, tables, chairs and everything else has to fit into one vehicle. An SUV or a pickup truck would be handy. I manage with a Jeep Wrangler but space is a factor.

Front of our tent set up for three readers in the front. The three folding chairs in the front of the tables are for clients.

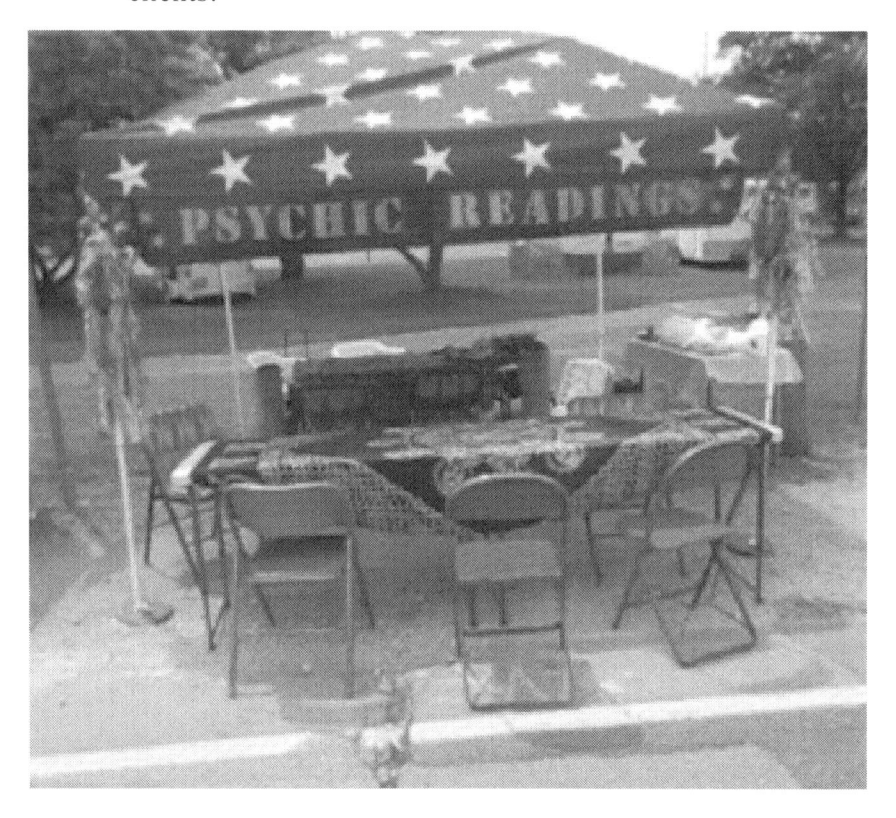

Festivals, Fairs and other big events 35

A look from inside the tent. Three readers all reading clients with curious bystanders waiting their turn.

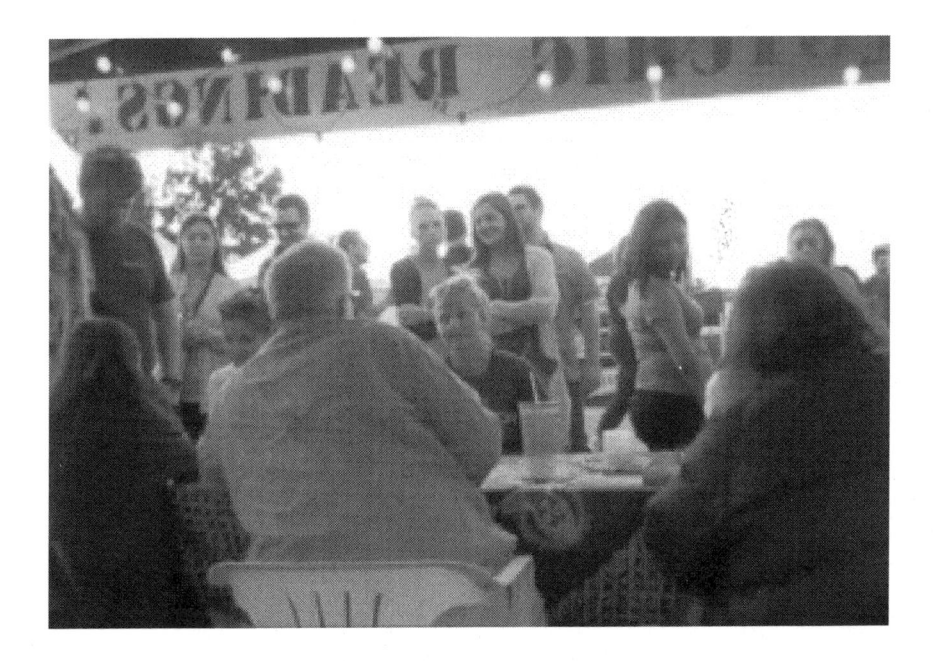

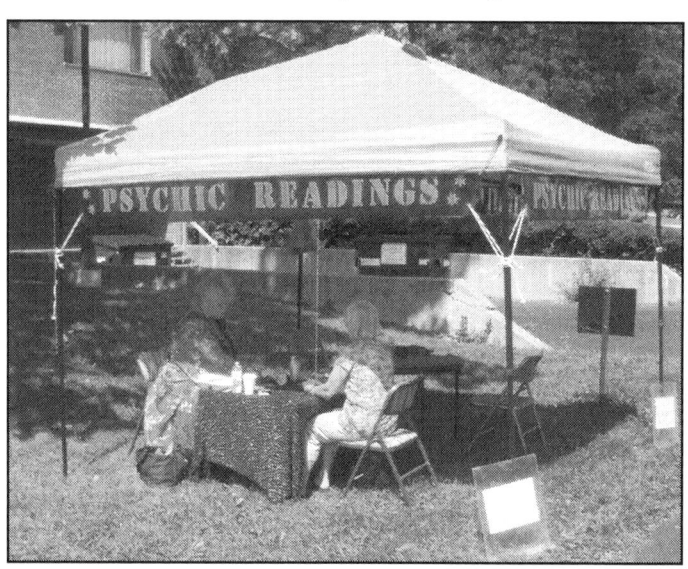

Picture of our tent. Lynda reading a client.

How fairs work:

Fairs usually go two, three, even four days. Thursday through Sunday is common. Hours will usually be from noon till midnight each day with Sunday sometimes being noon till 6pm. That's a rough guess. You probably won't be busy until 3pm or so on Friday and Saturday maybe even 6pm depending on the fair. Don't be discouraged. The night will bring out people looking for a reading. Noon to 6pm is slow except on Sundays which will just have a nice moderate flow most of the day. But on Friday and Saturday things usually get busy around 6pm. Six to midnight is when you make your money.

As a reader at events like this it will be important to make sure you watch your time. Setting a timer will help you with that. It also lets the client know when their time is up. A minute timer works well for this. A good way to end a reading is to wrap up the reading with what has been said as advice. *"So, we see that you need to do this and keep an eye out for this. It will come soon. This is what was seen to succeed on your quest,"* and things like that. Then, say, *" I hope you liked your reading."* If they don't stand up to leave, you stand up and wave the next person to your table. Keep it moving.

Setting up your table:
I don't like to have a lot of theatrics placed on my table like crystals and little decor. Nothing but my cards are on my table. This way, if I want to leave the table for awhile I don't have to worry about things being taken. Fairs are busy places. Expensive crystal balls and things like that are not a good fit for this type of setting. A few modest things are fine but don't over do it.

Getting started:
Go to a few fairs and see which ones you like close to you.
See if there is an INFORMATION booth somewhere on the fair grounds and ask who you might talk to about being a vendor next year. They will direct you to someone. Go during the day and that person will probably be on the grounds already. Go when they open up, not late at night. Late at night that decision maker will probably not be there. So go around noon time.

Price to be a vendor should be somewhere around $250 to $500 depending on the number of days the fair will be. This price range can vary a lot too depending on many things. But this is a good ball park figure. Most fairs run two to four days long.

Look for a Ferris wheel. If the fair has a carnival in it, it means the fair will be more than just two days. A carnival usually means a lot of people coming to the fair as well.

You will be better off if two of you work the fair together. Two or more readers works good. But one reader and a helper works, too, depending on the size of the event. Have someone there to help with things. Maybe a money taker? This way you don't have to worry about making change. It's nice to have someone there with you so you can take breaks, walk around the fairgrounds and not have to worry about leaving your tent unattended.

Making change:
I like to keep my prices at $10 and $20. 5 or 10 minute readings.
$25 makes it hard to make change. Everyone is going to give you two $20 bills and want $15 dollars change back. It gets to be a pain in the neck.

Two readers or more splitting the cost of a fair works well. It also is fun to have a group of you participating on the whole event. Have fun and make sure you hand a business card to everyone you read.

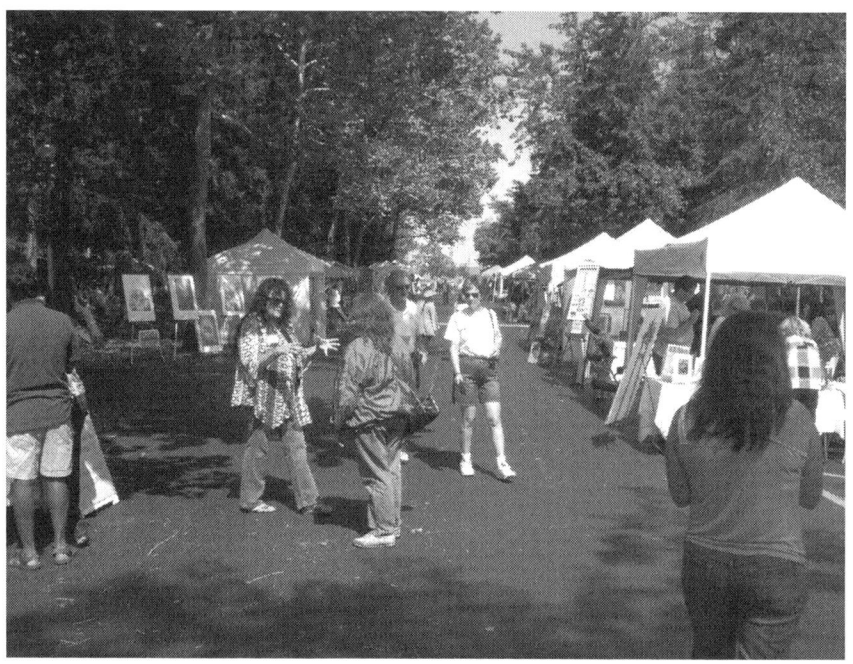

The Midway of a festival

Festivals, Fairs and other big events 39

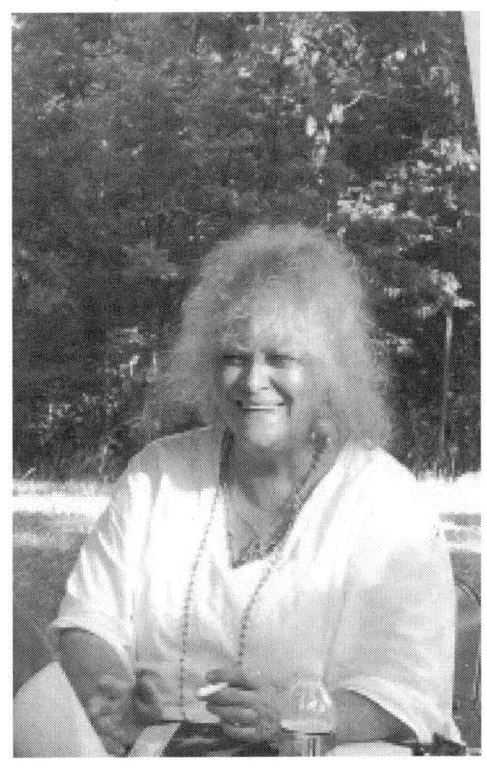

Lynda reading at a fair

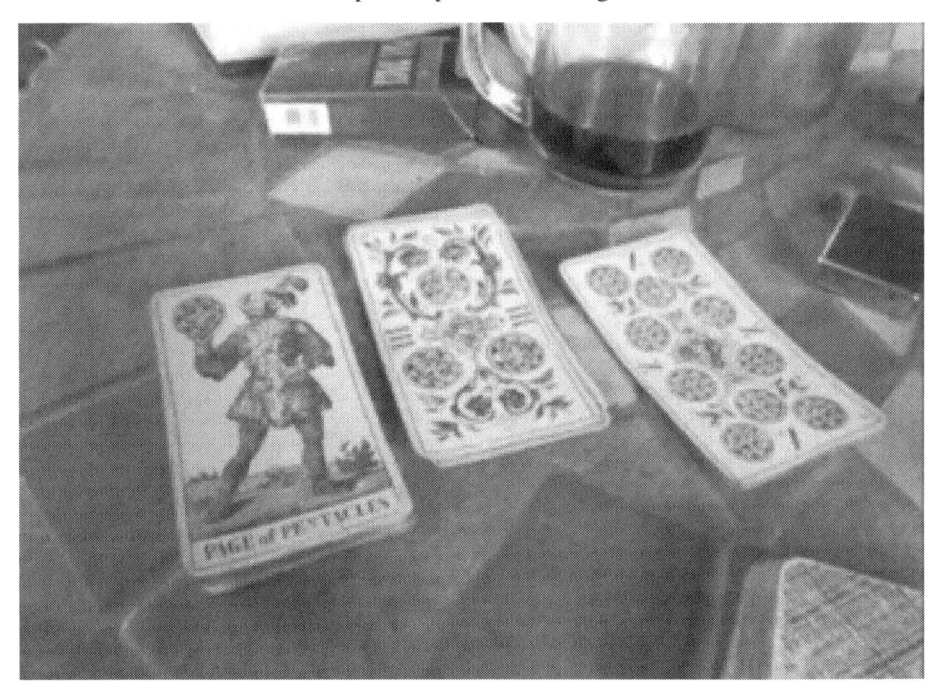

Back porch phone reading.

4. Phone Readings – A Key Asset

The internet came out around 1993. At that time psychic hot lines were big as well. They were advertised all over in tabloids. Lynda and I decided to look into doing psychic hot lines in 1996. At that time the rate was $4.00 a minute going to the psychic hot line service and the actual reader was only making around .25 a minute. We tried it for about two months and left.

We felt that the advertising of these psychic hot lines at the time was too deceptive and we wanted nothing to do with it. Many readers did the same thing at this time.

One thing we all discovered was you could do psychic readings on the phone successfully. They worked. This is when psychic phone readings really took off for the independent reader. Any setting we read in, we would let our clients know we offered phone readings just like the psychic hot lines did, only directly to us.

How to charge was still a challenge at that time. The internet was still very young and credit card charges online was still in its infancy. Anyone who wanted a phone reading would call us to schedule the reading, then send us a check by mail. Once we received the check, the check would have to clear at our bank. Then we would call the client to schedule the reading. Very involved process, but people did it.

We noticed that this phone reading thing had something to it. As the internet advanced, credit card charges online became more accessible.
By 1999 we had an online service and people could buy a reading instantly over the internet with us. This became very convenient for everyone involved.

Then the phone readings really took off. Today they are just a common purchase and no one really thinks it's a big deal to make online purchases.

I would have to say that half of my business is phone readings today. They are convenient for everyone involved and easy to do. And the reading is just as good as a face-to-face reading. I have clients that I haven't seen face-to-face in over ten years who call me regularly for phone readings.

The main reason I work at stores, do fairs, house parties, or any other face-to-face reading situations, is to meet potential future phone reading clients.

You will get business by being out there in the public, doing your readings here and there. You are doing that to drum up potential phone reading clients. That is how you get phone reading clients. Once they meet you face-to-face, doing future readings with you over the phone doesn't seem like such a bad idea to them anymore. They know you. They know how you read and then they feel comfortable doing future sessions over the phone with you. They are very convenient for them, as well as for you.

I would say that the phone reading today is the most important part of your business as a professional Tarot reader.

Most clients will initially say that they prefer the face-to-face reading. But once they have a few face-to-face readings with you, then they know you. They know what you look like. They know how you read. They just know you now. That is when they decide that they can do phone readings with you. Then, once they start, they will prefer to just call you. It's easier than getting in their car and driving somewhere to see you. And the readings are the same. Once they see that, you have a phone reading client.

Phone readings will be a large part of your business. At least that is the case with how things went for me. My strategy was to read in public settings to acquire future phone reading clients. Working in public settings allowed me to build my client base, which ultimately became a lot of phone readings – very few face-to-face sessions once we established knowing each other.

Much has changed over my time as a reader. This will continue and you will see changes in your time as a reader as well. Online readings are available today. Yahoo Instant Messenger and others allow visual communication now, too. I prefer not to do those types of readings, but you might want to look into them. They are probably going to become the norm as time goes on.

For me the phone readings work just fine. I might make money while having my first cup of coffee in the morning just by answering the phone and throwing cards down. Many people will call while driving on their way to work with some issue they want answers to. They are just sitting there stuck in bumper-to-bumper traffic anyway. So they think .....*Might as well do my reading now. I'm just sitting here stuck in traffic anyway.* It is just a very convenient way to read cards.

So from 1993 to 2018, twenty-five years changed a lot of things – for the better. I'm sure if you continue on as a reader you will see many changes in the next twenty-five years as well. You will see what is working and what isn't anymore.

And, you will follow the action and the money just like we did in our time. Have fun. We did and so will you!

The progression and interest in Tarot readings:
In the early 1970s psychic fairs were huge events. People were starving for this stuff and waited in line to get a reading from a few select psychics. Back then fate was considered a real factor and you would look at the cards to see someone's destiny. Readings were actually considered a little scary because of that perception.

The 1980s and 1990s were real big for New Age bookstores and many psychic readers were reading there. There were always psychic fairs each month and they were always packed full and very busy days for the readers.

The attitude for a reading was becoming a little more gentle in its approach to the future. Readers and clients felt that they had some control over their destiny and what could be accomplished.

Since then, the New Age bookstore is starting to fade away. The internet offers the online type reading but it doesn't seem to be going anywhere. Phone readings are now the big draw in this craft. That's where it stands right now.

Of course the face-to-face reading is still slightly more personal. But not enough to justify getting in traffic and driving somewhere. People just don't have time in their daily lives to drive in heavy traffic and waste time to get a face-to-face. If they already know the reader, they would prefer just calling for a phone reading.

Like all things eventually do, I'm sure this will be changing.
What will come for you is something even better! I just don't know what that is yet. But we will see soon enough. So keep an eye out for it.

Talk to other readers and see what they have to say as well.
Networking with other readers is an important part of the business.
Don't isolate yourself. Be out there and people will be talking about you.

Once you are established, if you add up all your business over the course of a year, half will probably be from phone readings.

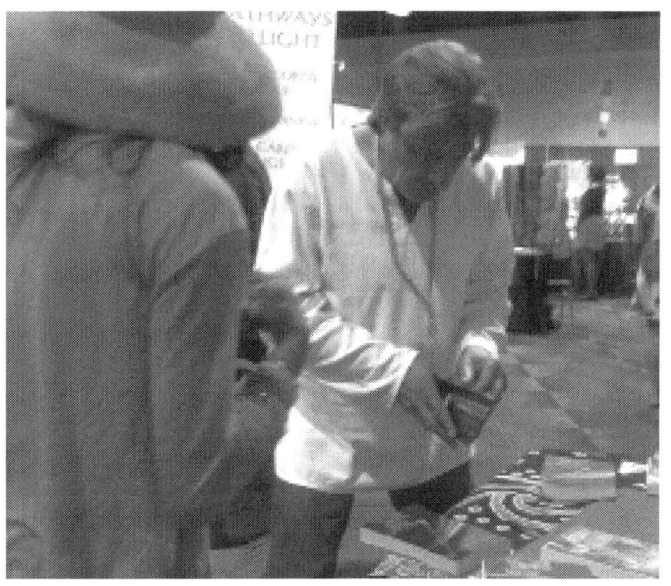

Reading and book signing at an event in 2015

5. About Reading Paying Clients

As you start to read professionally your readings will change from just curious Tarot readings to looking into serious matters. People will seek you out and pay you money because they have a need to find answers. They are stuck on some issue. They feel that their issue of concern is something that is out of their control and they are hoping you can give them ideas and solutions.

This is where you come in. A stranger comes in to see you, hands you money and now wants answers. Are you ready for that challenge? They need to walk away from your table with something they didn't have before they sat down with you. Some new insight. Direction. A plan. And if it all works, they will return. You have an opportunity to become their advisor.

Knowing the meanings of Tarot cards is helpful, but now you need to see tangible solutions to challenges that card definitions will only go so far with. The Tarot cards show you ideas. Choices. Options. You, the reader, will need to see those concepts in the cards.

One piece of advice I give to all my students to help them feel comfortable as a pro reader is to feel – *"I am here to help you find answers to your concerns."* Remembering this one important thing will help you feel a connection to your client as you read.

How do I solve this problem or achieve this objective is what's key.
How do I give this client some useful advice? That's why they are paying you. They trust you and confide in you.

I keep in mind a set of aspects that will help most any reading you will face. What is the real question and what is the client really looking to achieve? Why do they want this particular thing in their life? How can they go about getting what they want? When is the best time to take action on this goal?
Keeping those four elements in mind as you interpret the positions meanings in your card spread will help you find real purpose in the readings you give.

WHAT – WHY – HOW –WHEN

Answering just one of these aspects in some way that the client didn't see before could make the difference between their success or failure.

WHAT:
What is the real question? The underlying purpose of the question? Should we reformulate the question itself?
What is it the client is really trying to find? To accomplish? What is that one true thing? Many times this is not seen by the client clearly. Look into the real question.

WHY:
Why do they want this in their life? What do they feel this objective will give them? Will it give them what they really want? Or are they moving in a wrong direction for success?

HOW:
How is the best way to achieve this objective they seek to attain? What are they not seeing that can help them get this goal accomplished? What actions should be taken to create the best results to succeed in this goal? What actions need to be taken? What are they not seeing?

WHEN:
When is the best time to act on this objective? Does the client act now before opportunities are lost? Or is it best to wait for a more opportune time that will come in the future? Act now? Or have patience and wait for a more advantageous time in your favor yet to come?

More in-depth look into these four factors:

WHAT:
This allows us to really question the client's own perception of the situation they are in and what it really is. Many times a client can lose sight of the big picture. It allows us to question the client's own perception of their question itself. Is this what they really think it is?

WHY:
Why does the client want this? What do they feel it will bring into their life? Will it? Is there a better action to take to achieve the situation they want?

HOW:
Here we look at what we think will be the best way to achieve this objective. Is the client using everything they have at their disposal to help get this accomplished? Can things be done in a more effective way to enhance the chances for success? Is something being overlooked?
Any details not being seen that are important? Can we give the client an edge in this objective? An advantage not seen before they sat down with you?

WHEN:
Timing can make a difference. When is the best time to act can be key. Most clients are impatient and want to act now. If they wait, is there a time in the future that seems to give them a better advantage. Or is acting now in their best interest before opportunity is lost? When to act is key.

USING THESE FOUR FACTORS IN YOUR CARD SPREAD:
Keeping these four aspects in mind as you do your readings can bring out more potential in your reading. How can any of these four aspects be associated with the positions of my card spread? Can these four aspects be blended into the reading as I go through each position? Tilted or turned in some manner of meaning with these important aspects to success in mind?

Keeping these four aspects in mind as you look for answers in the reading will give you good results, no matter what spreads you decide to use.

They can help you see more purpose in the positions of a spread. Or maybe just fine tuning your position meanings with these four aspects in mind might bring out more insight into your readings.

You are trying to help a client and if you can feel their concerns, your readings will be accepted as sincere and worth the money you are paid.

Another factor to keep in mind is to stay in the light. You will do well staying away from focusing on revenge, bitterness, hatred, and any negative focus in your reading.

If your client wants to hurt someone else for what they did to them, you will be better off trying to get them to let it go and move on. They are better off to focus on healing themselves instead of hurting someone who hurt them.

Seeking revenge keeps them stuck in a low vibration. Happiness and clarity is best done by moving on and letting go.

Reading Medical Issues:

The only medical advice I give clients is for them to get medical attention. I am not a doctor and I have no business trying to predict medical conditions. Tell them to see their doctor. If they insist on knowing what you see in the cards say, *"I see you need to get your medical guidance from your doctor."*

Some people have emotional and mental issues that make their life confusing. Again, I stress to these people to see their doctor or to get professional counseling. Some clients suffering from paranoia will tell you they cannot trust their doctor or their family. Here you must try to guide them to understand that those people are not out to hurt them. They are coming from a space of concern and are trying to help.

I usually close the reading by saying, *The next time we see each other I want to hear that you are taking your medication and seeing your doctor.*

Some types of clients:
You will see differences in the type of client business you acquire. Here are some patterns I have seen over time.

The Internet Client:
This is a rare customer. People who have found you over the internet. Your website or some other place on the internet. These are usually phone readings, but occasionally they are a scheduled meeting for a face-to-face reading. They are usually just a one-time customer.

The Monthly Client:
These are people who make it a point to get a reading once a month no matter what is going on with them. These are usually short readings and are just update type readings for them. They are usually 15 minute or 30 minute readings and are very consistent, regular customers that can last for years. These types of readings are usually pretty casual and easy going. They are usually done over the phone.

The Comfort Client:
These clients just enjoy having someone to talk with about their affairs, good or bad. If they enjoy your advise and company, they are easy reads for you and will call anywhere from once a week to once a month. It is not uncommon for this type to enjoy hour-long readings whenever they can get them.

The Regular Client:
This type of client is currently going through some type of challenge. They will see you two to three times a week until the issue is resolved. This could go on for a week or as long as a few months.
Then, once that issue is resolved you won't hear from them until another issue in their life could use your counsel. Most sessions will be done by the phone with this client. Times will vary but are usually at least a half hour session.

Your Following:
As time goes on you will accumulate a number of Regular Client types who contact you with problems to solve. Help them find answers and solutions and they will stay with you for a long time. When a problem arises, they call you for advice and suggestions.

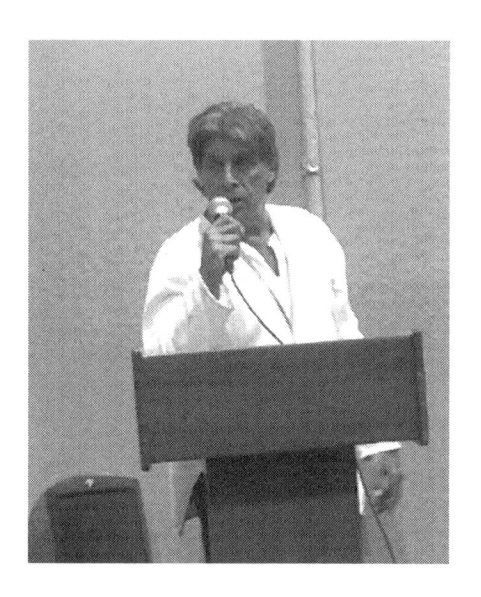

6. Little Bits of Insight

None of this is based on any facts. It is just patterns I have noticed over time so these are just things for you to keep in your pocket as you read cards.

At that first professional reading, you look at the cards and the card spread you have learned and you hope that you can do this. Did I learn enough? Your card spread might seem weak to you. OMG can I do this, or am I just playing with these cards?

Well you were just playing with the cards initially, but now it's the real deal. This is where you start to see that the card spread and the cards have a purpose, but that the real power is not in those things. The power is in the advice that the cards can show you.

Once you get to this point you start to realize that your intuition has its place in the reading, but so does your logic. They need to blend into each other for answers that are useful to the client.

Once you are given the responsibility to find answers you will use both logic and intuition together. The measure of one verses the other will vary with each reading you do.

So the number one thing to remember is that you are there to help this person find answers. That is your main purpose. To help them find direction. To help them means to feel them. To help them also means to think like them.

I feel I'm a card reader.
I think I'm a card reader.
Both statements are true simultaneously.

Ultimately, you are there to give them some piece of useful advice that will help them achieve what they seek. A strategy. A plan. A direction. Another important factor is you will see patterns with client issues. You will see patterns in client personalities as well.

The biggest strength you have is your intent. Not how well you know those cards. Your intent is what will make the reading good. Sure you will get to know those cards well in time. That's a given. But having that feeling that a person has trusted in your advice makes you want to help them. That is a strength you will have. You care.

One of the biggest challenges you will face as a professional is reading clients who you might not agree with. You may feel what they think is important isn't really that important. To you it isn't. But to them it is. You have to keep that in mind as you read others.

Having patience and understanding is key. You may think that what they want is trivial. But you are not that person. To read them well you have to feel their needs and hopes.

As long as they are not doing something that will hurt them, you need to help them at what they want to get. Even if you know that once they get this, it won't be as great as they think it will be. They have to find that out for themselves, although you can suggest and question them. As long as they are not hurting themselves or others, try to see their side of things.

If they want to deceive or wish harm to someone, then you can step in and tell them that isn't a wise move but otherwise their pursuits of happiness are theirs. Not yours.

DO NOT MAKE ACCUSATIONS WITH THE TAROT CARDS:
I feel it is good to remember that you are only telling them what you sense from the reading. That does not make it a fact. Therefore questions like "Is my husband cheating on me?" are not ones you can answer with a yes or a no. Focus more on ways to see how to improve the relationship. It is obviously strained in some way if she is asking a question like that. In time she will know the truth either way, on her own, about her husbands actions.

Do the reading as if her husband was sitting there with her at the table. He is not there to defend himself, and to accuse him of infidelity on the turn of a card would be wrong. Besides, if you say, "Yes. He is cheating on you," and then she finds out he wasn't, you will look really bad! You might even get a knock on your door from him wanting to know why you would tell his wife such a terrible thing.

What she really needs to do is find out what the problem is at home and look for a way to resolve it. You may be able to help her do that with your card reading. So the real question becomes, "What can I do about my marriage?"

Another example of these types of damaging questions would be, "Did this person steal something from me?" If someone asks a question like that to me, I just say I cannot answer a question like that with any accuracy. It wouldn't be fair to accuse someone. You can't accuse someone. But you can tell your client to protect herself and if she doesn't trust that person to back away from them, at least for awhile.

Remember that the things you say might have to be explained if you are called on it. I think it is wise to tell you not to downgrade anyone in your readings. That doesn't help your client anyway. Find something that will.

When you read professionally, you are not just a reader anymore. You are a kind of diplomat as well.

Patterns in readings of Love:
Probably the biggest topic on the reader's table will be love. You cannot force someone to love you. They cannot force themselves to love you, either. You cannot ask someone to do you a favor and start loving you tomorrow.

Like a favorite color, you cannot explain why a particular person is your personal preference. If your client loves someone and hopes that the feeling will be returned, there are certain things that person can do to give themselves the best chance for that to happen.

Telling them to express those feelings is good advice. Letting a person know you love them is good to do. But if things seem to be going slow from their partner – patience is key. No commitment. Remember, you cannot talk a person into loving you. You can only show them who you are and how much you care for them. Showing them who you are means being yourself.

It's a lot easier for someone to fall in love with you when you are just being yourself. Even with your imperfections, that is just who you are. Show who you truly are, and that you love yourself as well!

Optimism is key, too. Being up instead of sad or worried. Live your life and there is a good chance that person will want to live life with you. Dance, sing, cry, laugh, live! That is what is catchy to others.

People fall in love with other people who are happy with life itself. They want a part of that!

It's important that you know who you are. How can another person know who you are if you cannot show them who you are? And in order to show them who you are you need to know that yourself. Show them who you are.

Although looking good helps, your eyes and your smile are what count most. That and the touch of a hand are the things that make people fall in love easiest. The kiss will follow. Bet on it!

You can guide someone on how to proceed with a lover to give them the best advantage for that relationship to move forward.

You will also read many who are just lonely. That is a pattern as well. I tell people in that situation to have a relationship with society and they will meet other people that way. In other words, get out of the house; join clubs, special interest groups, your church and things like that.
Internet datelines seem to bring more confusion than actual success. At least that is my feeling. But getting out and getting involved with society in some way that interests you can be very beneficial in meeting someone new

Relationship patterns to watch for:
Separated but not divorced:
Being involved with someone who is separated but not divorced.
There is a good chance this person will end up back in their marriage after about one year's time of being separated. Your client should move slowly and not pressure the relationship. Her lover has a lot to process before starting another committed relationship. It can happen, yes – but it's a bad bet.

Recently divorced lover:
This person usually does not want to jump into another committed relationship for a few years. Move slowly and let this person heal and find balance in their life again.

Internet connections from another state or country:
Who's moving? Who's relocating needs to be established as the relationship becomes close. If from another country, it's a good idea to let them come here and get established before moving any further.

His job takes up all his time:
"His demanding career interferes with our relationship."
If you only see each other once a month, or even once every two weeks, the relationship shows signs of obstacles in moving forward. If he loves you he will find the time to see you no matter how much he is working. If he's breathing – he will want to see you. That's love!

Good signs in the start of a good relationship's first year or two:
Spending weekends together and maybe a visit during the week as well shows signs of the relationship moving along nicely. Now and then discussing plans of moving in together. Talking to each other everyday on the phone shows you are in each others thoughts as well. Good signs.

Other popular issues you will be asked to read into:
- Job promotions.
- Will I get this new job?
- Will I sell my house?.
- Will we have a child soon?
- Will I pass this college course?
- Will I be successful in my new business?

Logic vs Intuition:
I feel most of my readings are 90% common sense with a very important 10% intuition thrown into the mix. Intuition is like concentrated knowledge. 10% of intuition can go a long way. It's like salt added to the stew. Sure it's important, but too much will ruin the stew. Mix and stir gently. Logic and intuition blended together on realistic aspects of the questions being looked into will give you surprisingly good results.

Base the reading on logic and reason. Logic and reason is like the foundation to build the reading on. Then you can add a pinch of intuitive thought into that well structured reading.

Ultimately, I try to keep the focus of my readings on things I can prove at a later date to be true. I make predictions. "If you go this way - I see this happening." "If you go that way - I see that happening."

I stay away from things like past lives, spirit guides and soul mates. Why? Because I can't prove them. But if you want to know if you're going to sell your house by June. Now that I can look into. And in June we will know if I was right or I was wrong.

Some other thoughts:
- 80% of your clients will be women. (It used to be around 90% when I first started reading.)
- If you are reading a nurse, there is about a 25% chance she is married to a police officer or a fireman.
- Most people you read will be romantic type personalities.

Times of the year relationships are most vulnerable to break up:
- The Monday after a bad weekend.
- For college students, spring break is a peak time for breakups.
- Fourth of July weekends.
- First week of December.

You will have many unusual situations in your readings with clients, but most of them will be similar. The three items listed below are the most popular topics brought to your table:

- Finding love
- Career change
- Finding purpose in life

Relationship issues usually fall under three different categories:
- The relationship is just starting out and the reading is to see where it will lead.
- The relationship is established but is challenged at the present time.
- The relationship is stable but not moving forward in any direction of commitment. It's stagnant.

Infidelity:
Infidelity is usually caused by the relationship at home being a confused one. Like the song *"Do you like pina coladas?"* It is something that usually passes and the two end up back together. Only stronger than before if they can get past that rocky time in their lives.

7. Who am I?

Sun Tzu said that in order to master anything you need to know yourself first. (At least I think that's where I heard that from.)

So I will tell you what I'm all about in this craft of reading Tarot cards. I don't believe in spirit guides, soul mates, past life regression, or angels watching over me. I don't believe in curses, spells, possession or magic potions. I don't believe in astrology either.

I know many others in the craft who do believe in all of those things and we all get along great and respect each other. And they are just as good a reader as I am. I'm not saying these things don't exist. I'm just saying I choose not to believe in them.

I do believe in psychic awareness, spirits, auras, out of body experiences, and dreams showing you things. I believe in all of those things because I can say I experience them first hand.

I do not believe in fate. I do believe we have control over our destiny, at least to some extent. If you want to believe in fate, think of fate as the cards you were dealt in life. How you play those cards is your own free will.

With that kind of attitude we can look at our challenges in ways to avoid negative outcomes and encourage positive ones. If I see any negative situations in my readings I look for ways to deal with them. How can they be avoided? With positive ones, how we can continue moving in that direction.

Paying attention to how you think on certain issues will give you a clearer understanding of how you read for others.

There are things about the mind we just don't understand. But each decade we learn more. There are dimensions of our world, or even our universe, that we do not understand as well.

We cannot explain what life is or when it starts. At least not with any conclusive facts to prove our theories. We cannot understand what time is or how we can control it. Or even if we can control it.

My point is we do not know a lot about our universe or our place in it. We might feel we do – but there is still so much to understand.

I know that entities outside of the physical realm do exist. I have seen them first hand. I have not only seen people who have passed. I have seen people who are still with us, their astral bodies. I have also experienced astral projection myself. Out of body experiences. So I know first hand they are real. I have seen my future in my dreams. I see auras around other people. I have seen, heard and actually been touched by spirits. So I know they are here.

Do I feel they can harm us? Not at all. Why would they? They have an understanding about life that we could not comprehend being limited to just five senses in the physical realm. But we will eventually be there at the end of this physical journey we are all on.

We can see things around us if we pay attention and allow ourselves to open up. Our perception can go beyond logic and rational thinking.

I will share one of my experiences:
I don't want to give the impression that I walk around seeing all sorts of things other people don't see. But occasionally this does happen to me. When it does happen, I understand what it is.
So here I will share one of those experiences with you.

I walk by a hospital every night that's right on my block. One wintery cold rainy night around midnight I walked home and right across from the emergency room was a car parked where it shouldn't be parked. Next to the car was a woman who was obviously not right.

Her nice dressy clothes were torn. She was wearing a dark colored dress, and no coat. Her clothes were ripped and out of place on her. Even her nylons were trashed and she had no shoes. She was wearing heels earlier that night but not then.

The car she was standing by was a family member's car that she recognized and she was in a panic and lost.

Like she was looking for her family. She knew that car and was just waiting for her family to come out to it. I knew her body was in the emergency room and she was no longer with us. She just didn't know what was going on yet. And she clearly did not want to go into that hospital. She was confused, frightened and would rather wait outside for her family.

I saw, and clearly understood all of that in a split second of time. That's all it was. But she was there and I know if I had walked into the hospital I would have seen her family members there. How can I have known all that? All the details I saw? All in a flash of time? I'm sure she is in a good place now. But she left this world from a bad car accident. That I knew as well.

As you use the Tarot cards you will be opening up parts of your mind that you usually don't use in everyday life. Your intuitive mind opens up more and more as time goes on. The more you use it, the better it gets.

If you want to open up your psychic awareness there are many ways to do that. Actually, Tarot cards are probably not the most productive way. But they will do that if you use them. So reading the Tarot will improve your psychic awareness.

The good news is you will only open up to what you are willing to allow yourself to see. You will innately limit your perception to how much you think you can handle or want to know. No more than that.

I cannot control when things come to me. I cannot summon any spirit guides for counsel like many claim they can....in an instant. But then again, I am not interested in doing that.

But things are going to come to you. Don't worry, you won't be scared when it happens. You won't have time to be scared. It will come and go so quickly that it will be over before you can think about it. Fear comes from anticipation. Like in the movies....Don't open that door!!! No! Don't go in there!! AAAAHHHHHH!!!

When you are ready, they will just start to come to you.

Sometimes that will happen during your readings. Again, there are so many things we don't understand or can't explain but eventually we will know.

Maybe your generation. Maybe the next one. Maybe a little of each. What I do know is there are no evil forces surrounding your deck of Tarot cards. That's just a crazy idea.

You will find yourself having stronger connections with certain people and have a weak connection with others. This is usually because the strong connection is from people who trust you and are open. If you feel blocked by someone, they probably don't really trust you. Or they have something to hide and are concerned you will read their mind and discover it.

I tell people I can't read their mind and I cannot know anything they don't want me to know. That is their private place. Sometimes that helps put them at ease.

I don't have all the answers. I'm no different than you are. I have challenges and sometimes I'm not sure about direction either. Just like everyone else, I'm human. But I will try to help out my client sitting across from me the best I can. That's what a card reader does best.

After you cross my palm with silver that is!

8. Some Tarot Reading Stories

Over time you will acquire a number of readings that have stood out over the years. Sometimes you will see answers during a session that are just plain common sense to you. Other times you have no idea how you found the answers. They just came. Some of your readings might involved clairvoyance. Some are strictly grounded in the physical world.

As you read the Tarot you are using a part of your mind not normally used in everyday life, a part of your mind where imagination intertwines with logic. And imagination is the gateway to your intuition. So as you read the Tarot your psychic awareness will start to sharpen.

I thought it would be good to put a few readings in here that I have had over the years just to show you how readings can vary from one to another.

Here are a few examples from readings I can remember over time that have stood out, showing the different trains of insight that can come to you. Whether from the cards or not. Whether from logic or intuition or both.

The cat and the police officer:
I thought I saw a putty tat......I did – I did see a putty tat!

A woman came for a reading to the shop I was working out of.
She sat down and told me her situation. She was a police officer and she was hoping to get a promotion to lieutenant.

The promotion was under consideration and some interviews were already done. But waiting to hear if she got the promotion was driving her nuts. It had been awhile since she heard anything about it and she was concerned that maybe she was going to be passed by. She wanted to know what I saw in the cards.

As I laid out my cards I asked her a few questions like, *"How did the interviews go? How long have you been on the force? Are there others bidding on this position?"* The typical types of things that may effect the outcome.

As we were going through this reading I saw a black cat walk by me on my right. He stopped, looked at me and then proceeded to walk over to her.
(There are no cats in the store.) I stop the reading and I ask her "Do you own a black cat?" She looked at me, kind of surprised, as I asked this question totally out of the subject of her reading, and said, "I just put him down yesterday."

I asked "Was his name Jinxy?"

She said "OMG. His name was Mr. Jinx! And yes sometimes we called him Jinxy."

I said, "Well Mr. Jinx just walked over there to you right now."

Intuitive insight is usually recognized because of something from the heart. Not the material, but the emotional energy we can generate around us. Even though her reading was about the job promotion, what was in her heart was her pet cat, Mr.Jinx. That is why I saw him.

In her reading, I told her that her strong points seen by her superiors were her perseverance in her job as well as her determination. But her cat showed me she had compassion as well. I saw her being promoted more than once in her career in law enforcement. I never saw her again. But I'll always remember that black cat coming into the room. I'll also never figure out why I knew that cat's name.

But one thing I'm sure of – I'm sure today she is higher up in rank than she was when we had our reading.

The more you use the cards, the more your intuitive side will learn to work with your consciousness. Like any other thing you do, you get better at it as time goes by. Like a muscle, the more you pay attention and use your intuition, the stronger it will become.

Jesus Christ!:

Lynda and I did a monthly fair with about six other readers at a spiritual center for about 2 years. A young couple once came to me there for a reading that was very paculiar. First I read him. He was obviously not right. He had symptoms of Schizophrenia. He was very uncomfortable sitting with me. He told me he was Jesus Christ and was here to save the world. But the plan was to meet up with his guardian angel once he got here to Earth and get instructions on how to go about doing this. And he can't locate his guardian angel. This was very concerning to him because he said that the Devil was out to kill him before he could get on with this world saving stuff. It was important for him to find his guardian angel before the Devil got him. I calmed him down with the reading and told him he will find his guardian angel and all will be fine.

Then his wife sat with me. She explained the whole thing. He was a heavy using drug addict who had done damage to himself. He is in rehab. They were now divorced but he came back home after they released him from 3 months of rehab. He now saw a counselor once a week to see how his mind was improving. He was also medicated. I told her to give him time as long as he was trying to help himself. Eventually he would be able to function in society and leave the house.

The next month they came back. He urgently wanted another reading with me. She just shrugged her shoulders and brought him to my table to calm him down some.

He had the same story. Jesus Christ – here to save the world. Still can't find his guardian angel and the Devil is trying to kill him.

I calmed him down again.

Third month and again the same thing. There he was waiting to see me, first in line. He sat down and told me the same story with no changes in his situation. He was desperately looking for his guardian angel for direction and advice on how to save the world.

Then I remembered his wife told me he sees a counselor once a week. I said to him, "Do you have a counselor?" He said, "Yes. I do."

I said "That's your guardian angel! Do whatever he tells you to do and you will be fine."

He said "My counselor is my guardian angel?"

I said "Yes. He's been right there all along. Right under your nose. He will direct you on your journey. Listen to him."

I never saw them again.

There were no cards needed in those readings for him. Just some good advice coming from someone who he felt he could trust for advice.

I'd like to think he ended up OK.

Or maybe I really did read Jesus Christ and got lucky that his guardian angel really was his counselor! And he saved the world which is why we are all still here now! Cool!

I'll have some clout when I get to heaven myself. I can say I know the boss's son personally.

The Hot Dog Stand:

A woman came to me for a reading to see about her business. She was very nice, quiet and calm about the session with me. She wanted to know about her career. I was looking at the cards and I thought she serves the public. I said to her "Do you serve the public in your business in some way?" She said "Yes. I do." I felt that her husband was not involved with this business of her's so I said "Your husband doesn't work with you in this business does he?" She said "No he doesn't." I thought this was going along pretty good so far. I was really tuned into her and feeling more confident about our connection.

Then I said, "I see you going along well with this career of yours."

"Good." She said.

Then I went in for the kill. She said she serves the public. I thought of fast foods so I said, "I see you owning a fast food place. Maybe a hot dog stand. Is this true?"

She started laughing really hard. Then she said "No. But I am getting hungry." And she continued laughing.

I said "You don't own a hot dog stand?"

She said "No." Laughing wildly now. Which made me laugh with her.

I said "Well what is it then? Your business?"

She said "I'm a Congresswoman in the U.S. House of Representatives."

I lost it! I burst out laughing with her.
Surprisingly, the reading went well but we had a lot of laughs during our session. It was a good session. I told her she would keep her seat as a Congresswoman.

It was the last readings of the day for both Lynda and myself. Afterwards we went to a nice Italian restaurant right next door for dinner.

We ordered our meals and a glass of wine as we talked about our day. The next thing we knew the waiter came to our table with a bottle of the wine we were drinking and said this is from the table over there.

We looked at where he was pointing and it was that Congresswoman sitting with her friends having dinner as well. She waved to us. We waved back with a thank you.

I guess I did salvage that reading after all.

On the high seas:

Working as a house reader in a New Age bookstore and one day a young man came in for a reading with me. He was going on a job interview downtown for a position on a major cruise line. The job interview was held as a mass group and the recruiters would just ask a few quick questions to each of the applicants and then if you looked promising they would call you for further interviews. He wanted to know if he was going to get hired.

He was a young, single, good looking guy so I felt he had a good chance. I told him "Of course you are going to get hired."
He was happy to get my positive confirmation and left optimistic about his chances.

He came back a month later wanting another reading and said he did not get the job. I laid out my cards as we talked about what the interview was like. It was an auditorium full of hopeful applicants and the recruiters just walked by, asking a few questions, and then moved on to the next person. Very quick stuff.

My client was wearing ACE wrist support bandages on both wrists. I remembered he was wearing those same wrist support bandages at the last reading as well but I didn't think much about it at the time.

I asked him why he was wearing those on his wrists and he said he had sprained both wrists in a car accident so the doctor said to wear them for awhile. Then I tossed the Chariot card over. That card showed the Charioteer wearing armor like wrist guards on his wrists as well.

I asked him if he wore those wrist supports when he went on the job interview.

He said yes he did.

I asked my client if they were going to hold another mass interview again. He said, "Yes, they are." I said, "Good. Go again. And take those things off your wrist. They just show the recruiter confusion about you. Maybe something's wrong with you. So take them off your wrists. You have over a hundred people in that room with you who are not wearing wrist bandages. Who would you hire?"

He said, "I can't go back again. They would remember me from before."

I said, "Who cares. Go back and do it again. You'll get the job.
Did you wear a sports jacket?"

"No," he answered.

I said, "Wear a sports jacket, too."

He went back and did it again only this time wearing a sports jacket and not wearing those things on his wrist.

He got the job with a high end cruise liner touring the Hawaiian Islands. Young, single, good looking guy with no commitments working a cruise ship in the Hawaiian Islands. He would have never gone back and tried a second interview if it wasn't for his Tarot card reading.

Don't be afraid:

I worked a busy annual fair every year at the same place. Sometimes you will see a person you read the year before. A woman sat across from me for the first time and she seemed depressed. She was also very quiet and didn't talk much about herself.

The first thing I saw was the Tower card and I said to her, "Don't be afraid to have children." I didn't know why that is what I saw in that card but I did and I said it.

She didn't respond at all to my comment. I continued the reading and she was resisting the things I was saying to her. She wasn't cooperating with me at all. I covered career, relationship, and even family and health. Nothing was working. She said, "You're not telling me anything."

About half way through this reading I said to her, "What is bothering you? Can you tell me?"

She said, "I had a miscarriage and lost my child."

I said, "The first thing I mentioned in this reading to you was don't be afraid to have a child. It will happen if you allow it."

She didn't say much else. She was just down. She was not a happy person. She seemed disappointed with the whole idea of a reading with me and she left.

The next year we did that fair again. She was the first person booked to see me. She came to my table with a stroller with a little baby in it. She had a glow about her and her face was not the same face I remembered seeing last year, but it was her. She said to me, "I wanted you to see my child. Thank you."

There wasn't a dry eye in my whole deck!

Feeling lost:

I worked a New Age bookstore a number of years and you saw clients come and go. You get them through a rough spot in life and then they move on. That's what you do. And it can be very rewarding to you if reading the cards is in your blood. But sometimes it can also show a dark side of life. When you're a reader people confide in you. They look for hope and guidance. And sometimes things get by you. Details overlooked.

A young pretty girl around 20 years old came to see me about a love issue. She met a guy and she really liked him. She wanted to know how it would go. I told her it had good possibilities and to enjoy this exciting time in the relationship.

She came back a few weeks later and said that relationship went nowhere but she was involved with another. I kept the reading light and breezy and told her the same thing. Enjoy the time together and see where it leads. It looks good for you. I also found out that she was on medication and disability.

I could tell she had an emotional issue about herself for some reason. I knew she lived at home with her parents so I felt she was looked after and watched for. I hoped she would find a nice man in her life. She was a very pretty girl and had a lot of feeling in her heart. To me it was a sure thing to happen eventually.

Well she came to see me frequently. Always about a new relationship she was hopeful would get off the ground. And I always stayed in an optimistic tone about it to her. I wanted her to believe in herself and realize she had a lot to offer to someone. A heart of gold.

After about a year of this, I noticed she started to let herself go a little. Her hygiene and her appearance was really taking a hit. She just didn't seem to care about herself. How pretty she could be if she wanted to be. I also think she might have stopped taking her medication. But again, I knew she lived at home and was watched. I would ask her, "Are you seeing your doctor?" She would say yes as if nothing was wrong.

A few months went by without her coming in to see me anymore. I asked the owners of the store if anyone had seen her lately. They said, "We thought you heard. She committed suicide. Overdose."

That's when you realize you are not all that wise after all.
Why didn't I see something so significant and troubling in her. Maybe I should have seen that threat to her wellbeing.
Her sadness. Despair. Her feeling of hopelessness. Wanting to be loved by someone.

So remember that you won't see it all. Some things get by you. But you try your best. I'm sure there are words I could have said to her to make her feel better about herself. I didn't say them. And I will always wish I had said them.

Being a reader you will always remember the wonderful things you have done to change peoples lives. But you will also remember the things you didn't see – the things that got by you. It's just all part of it.

I've seen two situations where someone has committed suicide in the end. I can tell you this –neither one of them ever said, "I wish I was dead."

They hid their despair the best they could.
The only sign I can say I saw was they didn't keep themselves up in appearance. They didn't care what they looked like anymore. They didn't brush their teeth much either. They stop washing regularly as well. Maybe not that noticeable to others, but you can spot it if you pay attention. That is a red flag.

I'm sure a professional counselor would know more about those signs than a reader would. If you know one, ask them. To me, I noticed it in their teeth first – for some reason I can't explain. Their smile showed bad teeth. Not clean. Not sure if this was a clairvoyant perception or if they were just not kept up well. But their teeth looked wrong. Not clean. Something I noticed just for a second. A moment in their smile. A hint I guess.

But now if I see it again, in their smile, I will know where they are headed and try to steer them away from such despair.

An overly concerned but loving mother:

A woman came for a reading with her young boy about 8 years old. She told me he has nightmares. (Most children do.) She also said she knows his room is possessed with a demonic entity. (Most rooms aren't.)

She told me she has had a priest bless the room. A medicine man clear the room. She also hired shamans and other scary types to come and dance around doing ceremonies and other stuff with smoke and rattles and stuff like that in the kid's room!

I'm sure the kid's mother's dramatic actions probably scared the kid more than anything else. Inviting all these strange people to do things in his room like that. Most kids his age have nightmares. They are always sick with the mumps, measles, chicken pox, toothaches, earaches, and all sorts of stuff. Things like that make your sleep restless and can result in nightmares.

But she said that she can tell that the demon is still in there. She could sense it's presence. I'm thinking she is a *wack-a-do* but I keep quiet as she explains all this to me. She wanted to know if there was anything I could do to help protect her son.

I said, "Sure!" Then they sat together across from me.
I looked the kid in the eyes and he seemed OK to me. His mother was nuts. That's all. I threw a few cards down and then I told him that if he feels any demons in his room to tell the demon that it is not supposed to be there and it should leave.

Then I said, "Follow me," and brought them out to the store area and told him to pick out a stone from the display rack of various stones. He selected a *Tiger's Eye*. I told him that stone is a very protective stone and to keep it and put it under his pillow for a couple days.

I also told him if he sees any demons to tell them to come talk to me instead of bothering him. Tell the demon Vincent said so. They know where I live and will just leave you alone. They won't give you any more trouble. I'm sure the kid ended up just fine. The mother was nuts!

9. Other Professional Thoughts

Get a wall calendar:

After you have been reading professionally for a year you will want to look back and see how you've done. You will say to yourself – Wow! It's been a year already! Then you will try to recall all that you have done and what you still want to try to do yet. That first year will go by quick.

Do yourself a big favor. Get yourself a calendar. One you can hang on the wall somewhere with lots of space for each day of each month. Like a desk calendar.

At the end of each day write in the calendar any work you've done that day. Put names of clients down too. It doesn't have to be very detailed with phone numbers or who you read at the book shop you are a house reader at. I only put names of people when they are phone readings.

Example:

Sandy 30min. $50 phone reading
Bookstore $80 3 store readings
David 15 min $25 phone reading
Total $155

On days you had no work put a diagonal line through the square or an X.

Then at the end of the week, Saturday, total up all the money for that week from Sunday to Saturday and jot it along the side of the calendar next to that week. At the end of the month add up all the money you made that month and write down the total at the top. Then flip to the next month and start over.

At the end of the year you can go through it and see how many times Sandy got a reading with you all year. Same with David. You can see how much money the bookstore you are a house reader at made you this year.

Note any fairs you were at and how much money you made doing them. You can also see what months you were slow. What months were busy. This will help you prepare for slow months and anticipate the busy ones next year.

For me November and December are usually slow months. I think this is because people are thinking about Thanksgiving coming up. Family gatherings. December you have everyone thinking about shopping for x-mas gifts and money becomes tight quickly.

But then I think January would be slow because people get their credit card statement in the mail and it's huge because of all the x-mas shopping. But January is usually busy for me! Go figure. So who knows how people think. But at least you can track it with a calendar.

June and July are usually busy months for me. Not sure why but they are. Having a calendar will help you see how the pulse of it is for you.

Another good reason for keeping a record is if you have a discrepancy about a charge with a client. You might get a call from a client who is questioning a charge on her credit card statement from last month. She might have forgotten about a phone reading you gave her. You can simply go back to that date on your calendar and look.

If it is there, she had the reading.
You can say Yes. I read you for a half hour on the 15th. It's here in my records. This usually doesn't happen, but it can. I have had it happen maybe twice in twenty years but it was in my records so all was fine once the client got a confirmation that we did have the reading.

I always end the reading by telling my client, "I got you down for a half hour," (or whatever the time was) so they know up front.

I get my calendar each year at OfficeMax. It's a desk calendar but I hang it on the wall. The cost is under $10.

Always have your cards close by:
You never know when the phone is gonna ring for a reading. I have cards everywhere. I'm looking in my studio apartment right now and I have a deck in front of me as I write this book! One on the bookcase. Two on the table and two more on the shelf. Geez!

I have a few decks in my Jeep and if I get a call while I'm on the road I can pull over into a parking lot and read right in my car. I have a few decks at Lynda's here and there because I am over there every day as well. Usually no matter where I am sitting, I have a deck of Tarot cards within reach. It's just a habit. Just like my phone is always with me, so is a deck of cards even if I'm watching TV. They are there close by.

Scheduling your appointments:
I always try to read my clients as soon as they call me. If someone calls for a reading and you can't do it at the time they call, ask them if they are free later that day. If you know you will be available at 5pm ask if you can call them back at 5pm and do the reading then. Or ask when is a good time for them? Schedule something if you can. Your client will appreciate it and you don't lose the reading. Agree on a scheduled time and tell them you look forward to hearing back from them at that time.

The relationship with your clients:
Some of your clients will want to become friends with you.
You will have to ask yourself which do you want this to be, a friend or a client. They cannot be both. If you make them your friend that is fine. But remember that they are no longer a paying customer. Now they will be calling you to "talk" as your friend. You can have a good working relationship with a client, but that is not a friend.

Don't go to a client's house for social events, birthdays and things like that. Keep the relationship client-based. You spend time talking when they are in session with you. Not socializing. Socializing is for friends and you don't pay friends to talk with you. It is a common tendency for clients to want to be your friend. It seems like everyone wants a psychic for a friend. Just keep that in mind as you read.

We all want something for nothing:
It's human nature to want something for free. You see it advertised everywhere. FREE ESTIMATE! FREE BROCHURE!
FREE LARGE BEVERAGE WITH MEAL! Your clients are no different than anyone else. If they can get free advice from you they will take it.

You might have a client call you and tell you they just want to ask a quick question. You need to respond to that type of approach with "Do you want to schedule a reading?" They might say "Well I just have a quick question to ask." Tell them they need to schedule a reading. They might say "I just need a minute of your time."

Tell them your minimum charge is $25, 15-minute reading. But if the reading is only 2 minutes long it is still charged as a 15-minute reading. Minimum $25. If you give in to them they will call you constantly all day long with another quick question and the phone won't stop ringing.

You have to honor your work. I tell them that as well. Tell them they need to honor your work and this is what you do for a living.

Don't TEXT with your clients:
Texting is for a quick message and if your clients know you will answer their text message they will have numerous questions that they will text message you with instead of scheduling a reading with you. Things like "He just called. Should I call him back?" Don't answer text messages from clients. Or if you respond to a text message at all just reply with "Sorry. I don't text. You need to call me." Then when they call, you can tell them to schedule a reading.

Collect before you read:
Anytime you are reading in a situation where you collect the money directly from the client it is a good idea to collect the money before you start the reading. The reason for this is if you get busy and are reading one client right after the other you could forget to collect your money for one or more of them.

I never put a card on the table unless I was paid first. It is just part of the routine. This way I don't have to try to remember if I charged that last reading. Another reason for this is to make sure that they have the money on them. They might not, or they might only have a $100 bill and need change. Tell them they need to get change and come back unless you can make change yourself. Get paid first. Then read.

If you are doing a house party or a fair, the price is usually set.
Like $20 – 10-minute readings. These are the types of reading situations where it can be easy to forget collecting your fee on a few of your readings. It can get busy. You start the reading by saying hello and ask their name. Then say, "I need $20 before we start."

Exceptions to this are phone readings and regular clients that you know well enough. You know their credit card will work because you have processed it in the past. Another situation where collecting is not an issue is when you are a house reader at a store. The store collects the money and pays you at the end of the day. Not the client.

The Tarot Cards Themselves:

A Tarot reading is all about predicting a correct answer or strategy to achieve some goal a client wishes to accomplish. Wanting to accomplish means in the future. This is why you are paid money for your insight.

So how do we get that insight from a pack of cards? Many will say that the Tarot taps into our higher self. Or maybe our collective consciousness. The symbolism seen in all of these various decks, although not consistent with each other, is key to our awareness using the Tarot. None of these theories can be proven. Some of them don't even make sense. We have thousands of various style Tarot decks out on the market today. All of them have different symbolism to them.

The most authentic Tarot deck still in circulation today is the Tarot of Marseilles which looks nothing at all like the Tarot decks out there now. But that deck is probably the first deck used for divination with Tarot cards. The first real records we have of divination with the Tarot are from the late 1700's, France, and the Tarot of Marseille was what was available at that time.

Understanding what it is you are doing with these cards helps your readings tremendously. The Tarot is an idea generator. The application of a Tarot card reading allows us to see things about a question that we didn't see before we sat down with the cards. It gives us new ideas about what we seek to accomplish. Whatever that may be. It allows us to apply a way of thinking that cannot be achieved with conventional thought. And it works. But not because of the symbolism found on a particular Tarot deck.

It works because it is used as a very effective creative thinking technique. Our mind naturally thinks this way if we allow it to. Today this creative thinking technique is identified and clearly understood by cognitive science as Conceptual Blending.

So today why the Tarot cards work as an effective way of finding answers to future objectives can now be explained with conclusive facts for the first time in its history. The Tarot cards are no longer mysterious.

But the mind is still something we don't know a lot about.

We are explorers:

It's vast. It's unknown. It's unexplored territory.
Can we really see into the future? Or do we have the ability to create it ourselves? What is time? Can we explore time itself?
What about Intuitive thinking? Psychic Awareness? Clairvoyance? Astral Projection? Are they real?

These are subjects many people recognize as a reality.
They know they exist. They know things and see things that can't be explained. Just like knowing your favorite color. You just know it – with no rationality behind why.

Some day cognitive science will be able to explain these mysteries of the mind. They will have an understanding that is not here yet. They will have boring systems and procedures in place with logic and reason behind why this is what it is.

You might even be able to get a college degree on Intuitive Thinking. Learning all about how it works and why. Knowing that part of the mind. About time itself. It will all be figured out and explained. Knowing and memorizing all sorts of rules with no more to wonder about.

Those people in the future will look back at the Tarot readers today as explorers, pioneers in a world that had only vague direction. No real rules. What an exciting time. They will say, "Can you imagine what is was like for them? The wonder they experienced on their journey?"

Pioneers into an unexplored realm of discovery.
That is what the Tarot reader today will be seen as in the future. An explorer into unknown regions of the mind. Stray cats would be an appropriate way to define this curious lot.

That is the journey you are about to take. You are embarking into realms we know very little about. But we see hints of reality. Hints that can't really be denied. Conquistadors of the mind. Not knowing what's ahead, but having a thirst to find out. And making a living with the little insight we have to work with. You are leading the way. A footloose explorer.

10. How to Approach Professional Readings

Most of those just starting out feel that they are not supposed to ask questions to the client. You are just supposed to know things. This type of thinking can force the reader into a guessing game. Don't go there.
Get as much information about their issue as you can. Don't be afraid to ask questions.

If they are paying you money, believe me they will tell you what they seek to know. Your answers are what you are paid for. Not guessing their questions. They already know what is on their minds. They need answers. You are being paid to tell them what they don't already know. Not what they do already know.

As a professional you will get most clients coming to you with a specific concern. They are paying you money because they want answers to a specific challenge. You are charging a fee and they have specific issues they want addressed. The people are paying you to find answers and they will have no qualms telling you about their situation.

This allows you to use the time in the reading to find useful information for the client instead of feeling around trying to find out what the issue is.

Ultimately we want the client to walk away with some useful insight that they did not previously have before they sat down with you. You are a problem solver. An answer finder. Although intuitive insight will come to you during many of your sessions, you are not a carnival act. Your goal is to give them the best advantage to accomplish what it is they seek.

So ask questions. Why are you here? Are there any issues of concern you are trying to accomplish? Relationship, career, goals for the coming year?

They will tell you what is going on. Then you can get to work.

First I look at the question in a rational way. Then I build from there going into what the cards are telling me. Whether through intuitive insight or not. I am looking for ideas that were not seen before we sat down.

Intuitive insight is like fishing. You can't chase the fish. You set the situation and wait for a bite. It will come and the more you do it, the better the situation and setting you create.

You will start to see what works for you. The things you put on your table. Maybe the lighting. Incense, candles. And yes, a particular Tarot deck.

It's ritual. What is ritual? Location, specific items and procedure.
Just like the fisherman has ritual. His favorite rod and reel. Tackle box. Maybe certain things to wear like a particular hat. A certain time of the week and that secret fishing hole he likes best.

Think of it in the same terms. You're fishing for insight. And hope you get some bites today. If you're a professional, your chances are better than if you're not a professional. You know where to look and what to look for.

It's as simple and as complicated as that.

My advice is to move slowly on your new endeavor. As they say, "Don't quit your day job." Start by reading on the weekends at a bookstore or coffee house. Maybe book a neighborhood festival and see how it goes. Then after you get your feet wet – take the plunge and go all the way!

You will know when the time is right for you.

The going rate for my services in 2018:
This will give you a ball park figure on how much to charge for your wonderful services. It seems to be roughly the going rate for the other readers and stores I work with as well.

Many of the New Age type bookstores you may read in will already have set prices for what they charge in the store. This will give you a good idea of what you can charge outside the store as well.

Today I read in a few stores. One store has four options for clients to purchase.

- 15 minute reading – $25
- 30 minute reading – $50
- 45 minute reading – $75
- 60 minute reading – $100

I receive 70% of the purse and the store gets 30%.
Most stores take anywhere from 25% to 50% of the purse.
I get paid cash at the end of each day. The store will advertise you as a house reader on FaceBook and other medias. The store makes all the appointments.

The second New Age bookstore I read is a little more pricey than most and they only offer two options.

- 30 minute reading – $75
- 60 minute reading – $150

I receive 50% of the purse and the store receives 50%.

My own prices outside of stores are the same as the top list.
- 15 minute reading – $25
- 30 minute reading – $50
- 45 minute reading – $75
- 60 minute reading – $100

If someone calls you directly and wants a reading with you at the store, tell them they need to call the store and see what is available. You won't know that information until you go there. The store keeps that schedule.

However, if any of your clients you initially read at the store call you directly and want a phone reading with you, it has nothing to do with the store and you process the reading through your setup PayPal or whatever you are going to use. The store gets nothing from you and you keep the whole amount of the reading. It has nothing to do with the store at that point and is all yours to keep.

Stores understand that and there should be no problem with that type of setup. If there is...find a different store to read out of.

How to build a client base:
This is how you make a living now. So any readings from any client done in the store, the store takes their percentage. Any reading done outside of the store is all yours to keep.

The client will decide what works best for them. If they want to go to the store...buy some candles, incense, and get a reading... so be it. If they just want a phone reading, they call you directly.

You will end up with clients who see you in both scenarios. Sometimes they come to the store. Sometimes they call you directly.

Make sure you hand out your business card to everyone you read at the store. I tell the client, "If you would like another reading with me, I'm here at the store every Wednesday and Thursday and you can call the store to schedule another appointment. Otherwise you can call me directly for a phone reading anytime you like. I take Visa and Mastercard right over the phone. Here is my card. You can call me anytime. I'm here for you either way."

Anyone I read, I make sure I end the reading by telling them that if they would like another reading with me, I read over the phone and take Visa/Mastercard. You can call me anytime and set up an appointment. Here is my card. This holds true for house parties, festivals, stores I read out of. Just any readings I do.

You can see how phones readings can start to build up a client base. You meet people – You read them face to face – You let them know they can call for another reading anytime – Then the phone rings. Once they start calling you on the phone for their readings it can become a regular thing for them to do. Maybe once a week, maybe once a month, maybe two or three times a week. It depends on the client and what they are currently going through in life. And you will be there for them.

These become your regular clients. Some will be with you for many years. You become their reader.

The reason you read out of bookstores, coffee houses, festivals or any other public place is to build a client base. They can see you face to face and then feel comfortable doing other types of readings with you like over the phone. That means calling you up directly. You are out there reading in public scenarios, building a client base which ultimately means lots of future phone readings.

The phone reading client is where it is. That has been the case since the late 1990's. Will it change some day. Of course. Something better will come along, but for now it is still the best source of income in this line of work. Phone readings from a steady client base. At least that is my opinion.

The internet has great stuff that can work well for you too. Things like Google AdWords will get you readings. But the regular steady client only seems to come from initially meeting you face to face. Networking by working in stores doing festivals and things where people can really meet you in person, up close and in their area. Being local. Google AdWords can't do that. So get involved in some places where you can be out there reading in public.

11. Reading the Tarot Fluently

One of the things I teach in my classes is an exercise I feel is something you can always improve on. That is reading the cards fluently. Talking the reading through as you are laying the cards into each position. Creating a story where each card fits with the previous card as you are placing the cards into each position. I call this reading fluently and is a nice way to start the reading before going into the reading with more detail.

This looks quit impressive when you get it down pat. It also forces you to use your intuitive side instead of just memorizing card meanings. You will surprise yourself as to what you will see in the cards using this technique.

A good way to start practicing this technique is to use the Three Card Spread. It is just three positions being *Past*, *Present* and *Future* about a specific issue being looked into. Think of any topic and lay the first card down and speak what you see about the *Past* on this issue. As you are talking, lay the second card down and go right into what is seen in the *Present* on the situation without any hesitation. Then throw down the third card and effortlessly start talking about what is seen for the *Future* on the issue of concern.

Then come up with a finishing statement combining all three. This is all done in about one minute's time.

Past   Present   Future

Practice this and I feel you will like it. As you get comfortable doing the Three Card Spread move on to try doing this with maybe a five or seven card spread like the Horseshoe Spread.

The Horseshoe Spread

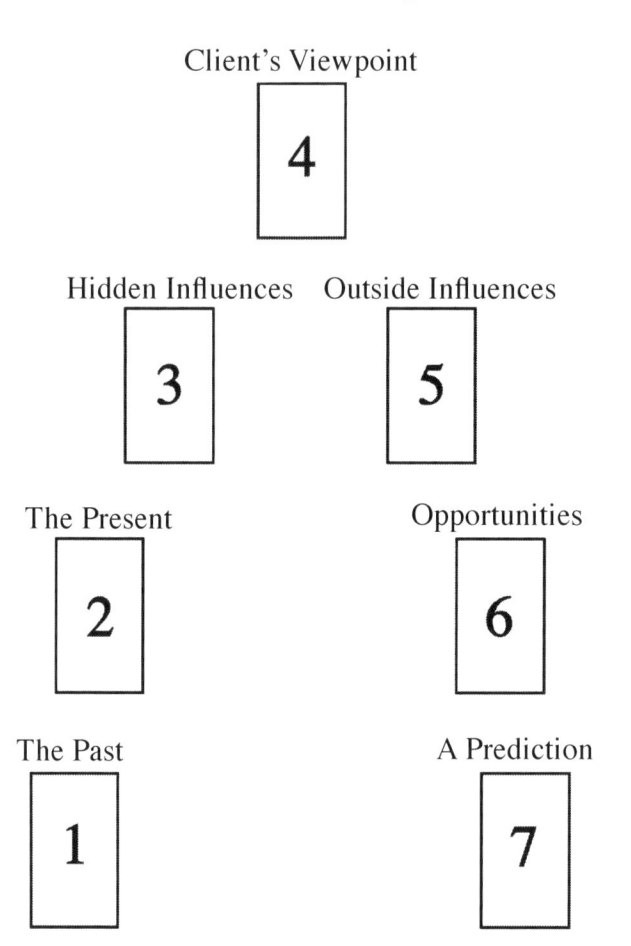

Client's Viewpoint
4

Hidden Influences Outside Influences
3 **5**

The Present Opportunities
2 **6**

The Past A Prediction
1 **7**

You will come across both a five card and a seven card version of the Horseshoe Card Spread from different sources.

After awhile you will get comfortable with that many cards. Then try doing it with the Celtic Cross which uses ten positions. When you can read a Celtic Cross fluently without any hesitation as you lay the cards into each position it is an impressive sight to see being done.

Your clients will know that you are very familiar with the Tarot cards once they see you read fluently.

The Celtic Cross

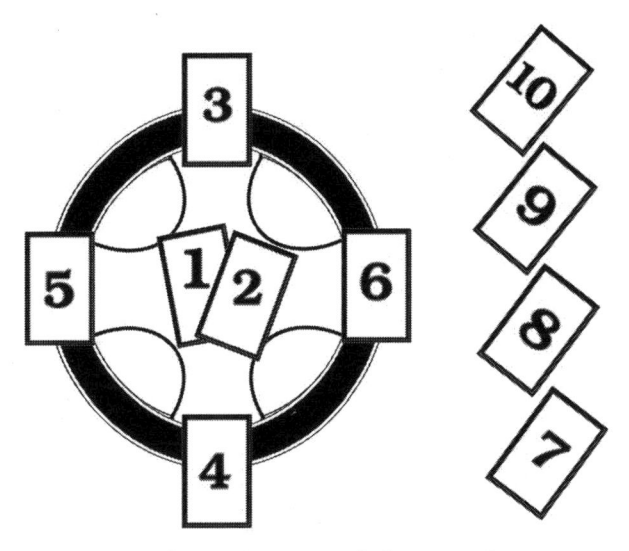

Position 1 & 2 • Aspects of the question
Position 3 • Client's current position

Position 4 • Client trying to accomplish
Position 5 • An asset of the client
Position 6 • An opportunity to come

Position 7 • The client own view point
Position 8 • When to act
Position 9 • The ultimate goal

Position 10 • A prediction

One other thing I feel is worth mentioning about reading fluently. The way you handle the shuffle or rearrange the cards during your readings.
Tarot cards are usually large cards. Most readers are women. Women usually have smaller hands than men do and it might be difficult for you to shuffle the cards because of this. That can make things appear awkward as you are reading.

If this is true, I would suggest just taking the deck and fanning the cards out on the table in an arch pattern from left to right instead of shuffling the deck. This looks very impressive when it's done well. Then you the reader, select the number of cards needed to do the spread from the fanned out deck one at a time.

It's just a minor detail I thought I would bring up. I know many fantastic readers who just can't shuffle Tarot cards and they still do well as readers even with a clumsy shuffle.

Another option is to purchase the *Mary Hanson Roberts* Tarot deck. The artwork is kickin and its size is smaller than most other Tarot decks.

12. Why the Tarot Works

Understanding why the Tarot is an effective application to see ideas not seen before you sat down with the cards will give you an advantage as a reader. It frees the Tarot up for you in ways most other readers haven't seen yet. It takes you away from rigid and limited procedures and meanings the cards can bring you. It will take you out of paint-by-numbers type readings and open up significant awareness into what is really being accomplished.

The reason I started writing about the Tarot in 2012 was because I saw what is truly being done in a card reading. The reason it is so successful.

Today the application of a Tarot card reading can be seen as what is known as a creative thinking technique. Specifically, a Creative Thinking technique known as Conceptual Blending. Google *Creative Thinking techniques* and *Conceptual Blending* and you will see what you read about is applied to the same application as the Tarot card reading.

The procedures are identical. They are also for the same purpose. To see answers we didn't see before. Answers for objectives to be accomplished in the future. In other words, to predict an outcome.

For centuries the Tarot cards have been stereotyped as mysterious. Unexplainable. That mind-set is still very strong, but today cognitive science can explain this imaginative and intuitive technique with conclusive facts.

Today the Tarot card reading would be defined as a Creative Thinking technique commonly known as Conceptual Blending. This is why it is so effective in finding answers and solving problems pertaining to the future.

Understanding why the Tarot works also gives you a view of why the cards show you answers. Each Tarot card in the deck can give amazing insight into elements of any question they are positioned with. Whether a card is placed into position 5 on your spread or position 3 on your spread makes no difference. All the cards will give you some type of insight and answer no matter what position they are placed in.

Each Tarot card's meaning is fluid, not rigid. The insight you see in a particular card will change from one question to another. Each card can help you find answers into whatever issue you are looking into at the time.

It is a universal tendency to fragment a question into separate parts. That is a necessary step for any analysis to be made. A card spread is your question broken apart into these separate parts.

The card spread represents elements of a question being looked into. Each card position is an element of the question being looked into. That is the purpose of a card spread. To break your question apart into sections to be looked at individually. The card spread is the question broken apart into useful elements of concern to look into.

The Tarot cards placed into those positions are meant to be used as possible answers or solutions. The randomly placed Tarot cards are used to spark new ideas to the reader as answers. The reader's mind forces itself to make associations between the Tarot card and the element of the question it is placed with. To connect the dots. That means a Tarot card's meaning will shift from one reading to another.

Your mind will conceptually blend a Tarot card's meaning to the position it is placed with in a way that will fit and make sense to what we are looking into. This type of thinking process cannot be achieved with conventional thinking. It uses your imagination, and imagination is the gateway to your intuition.

Conceptual Blending is a creative thinking process that involves blending two or more concepts in the same mental space to form new ideas. Like blending a random Tarot card with an element of a question known as a position in a card spread.

One of the elements has to be chosen randomly and blended into the other for meaning not seen before. The interpretations are usually done by making metaphorical analogies.

This type of thinking process today is data-driven. It is also being used in the study of artificial intelligence.

The centuries old Tarot card reading can now be seen as a very old form of artificial intelligence. My work goes into this new understanding in more detail.

With that said, I will end by saying we are just scratching the surface into the depth of intuition and psychic awareness that Tarot readings can create.

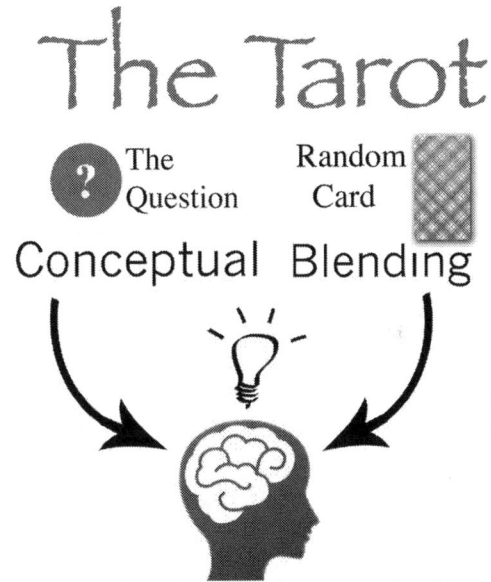

The Tarot

The Question — Random Card

Conceptual Blending

Scholarly interest in creative thinking is recognized by engineering, psychology, cognitive science, education, philosophy, technology, sociology, linguistics, business studies, song writing, comedy writing, economics, and many other disciplines.

It seeks deliberate, structured applications of thought to stir new and innovative ideas, solve problems and answer questions. Questions for things to be done in the future.

In other words...to predict.

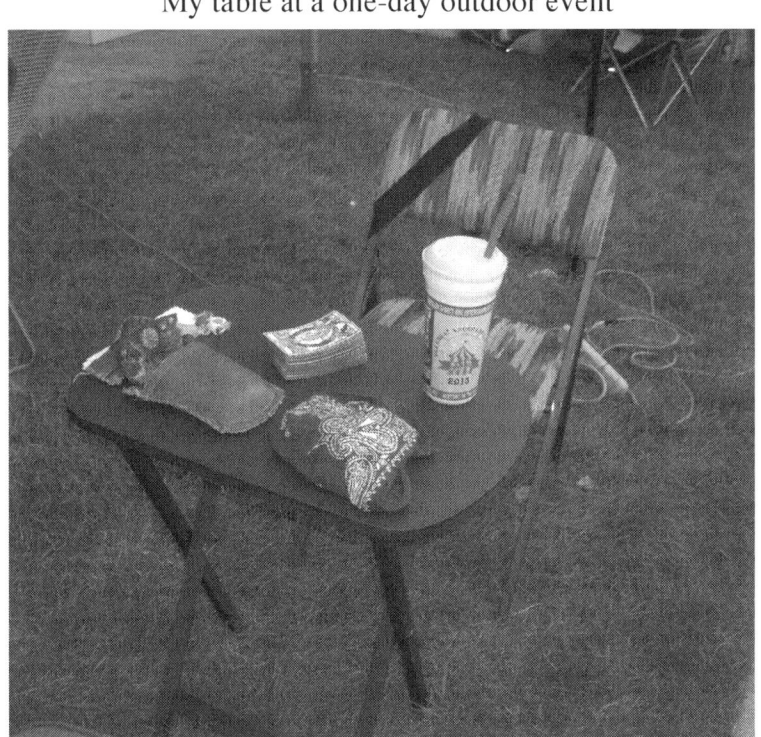

My table at a one-day outdoor event

Are you ready?

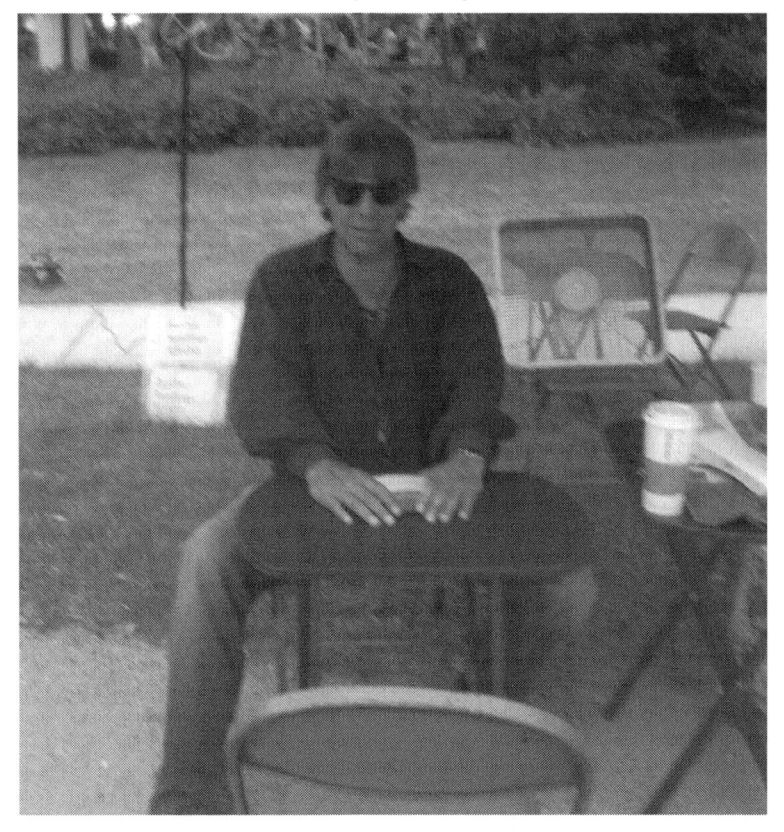

Other books by Vincent Pitisci.

Genuis of the Tarot – A Guide to Divination with the Tarot Cards

The Essential Tarot – Unlocking the Mystery

Coming in 2018!
Radical Tarot – Breaking all the Rules

Available on Amazon.com and Barnes and Noble.

More information on Vincent Pitisci can be found on the internet.

Made in the USA
Columbia, SC
25 March 2023

....4-138213688-LFNW7SJZ

_flushfilters --end-- }

errupt-- }

upt-- --disableinterrupt-- ( )
ch-- --put-- --clear-- }

Made in the USA
Columbia, SC
25 March 2023